"The treatment of chronic musculoskeletal pain has long been limited in scope and success. Fortunately, new treatments are now available which are simple, safe, and effective for a wide variety of chronic problems. This book outlines, through clear descriptions and numerous clinical cases, four of these techniques which are on the forefront of orthopedic medicine.

"Of these treatments, classical prolotherapy has the longest and most robust research and clinical basis. It provides the foundation for the other therapies: platelet-rich plasma, perineural superficial injections, and autologous stem cell injections.

"I recommend this book as an excellent informational guide to the many patients with chronic musculoskeletal and joint problems, as well as to physicians, in considering what is becoming first line therapy in the treatments of chronic pain."

—**Jeffrey J. Patterson, D.O.,** professor of family medicine, University of Wisconsin, and President, Hackett-Hemwall Foundation

"Regenerative Healing for Life reveals a biologic treatment revolution here today. The traditional orthopedic paradigm is failing many patients. I urge anyone with an injury to read this book, particularly if you are contemplating orthopedic surgery."

—**Christopher J. Centeno, M.D.,** co-founder of Regenexx and international expert on regenerative healing

"Through my experience with cancer patients, I have discovered what the authors of *Regenerative Healing for Life* share: The body has an amazing potential to heal. We physicians need to learn from the experience of successful patients and not be limited by beliefs created by our narrow information and training. Read on and learn from the success of others. Then incorporate these lessons into your practice and life."

—**Bernie Siegel, M.D.,** New York Times bestselling author of *Faith, Hope & Healing* and *A Book of Miracles*

"Before I met Dr. Shiple, I was ready to give up triathlon racing. With his help and several PRP treatments, not only was I able to compete, but I finished two Ironman races and successfully participated in the 2012 World Championship in Kona, Hawaii."

—**David Spartin,** senior vice chairman of MBNA and Ironman triathlete

"When stopping isn't an option as an athlete, Dr. Shiple and prolo or PRP are the only option!"

—**Tracey Greenwood, Ph.D.,** IFBB fitness professional, associate professor of exercise science, Eastern University, Department of Biokinetics

"I had plantar fasciitis. The pain was so severe that I couldn't walk. I had a series of four shots a month apart...after the first shot it was 90 percent better. I could not believe the relief I had. By the fourth I was totally pain free...now I can walk barefooted on the beach again."

—**Dorothy Butscher,** school secretary

"The prolotherapy has helped immensely...after every treatment I felt better. I haven't felt this good in five years."

—**Kara Feeney,** interior designer and nutrition student

"I had extreme pain in my feet for over a year. I went to every doctor in the book and they diagnosed me with all kinds of problems and nearly every one of them had me in a wheelchair. I was in a terrible situation when I went to Dr. Shiple. Now I'm cured. I owe my ability to walk to him. He is a real one in a billion."

—**John C. Oliver,** contractor

"Where I was to where I am now is night and day. I would absolutely recommend prolotherapy. Dr. Shiple is truthful and not afraid to try new things. He has a lot of courage. If he doesn't like something, he isn't afraid to change it. He makes his own destiny."
—**Jarrod Schoffler**, retired Marine Corps captain

"Dr. Shiple has risen above any and all expectations of other doctors. He is really just that good. Prolotherapy and PRP aren't masking agents; they are a rehabilitation process.

"PRP and prolotherapy saved my life. I am running again within moderation, both cross-country, in the woods, and with obstacles. I am also swimming and aggressively mountain biking. I would go to Dr. Shiple's office on Monday and clean the floor with a toothbrush and make it spotless. That is how much I support him and Marlise Wind in their vision to educate others."
—**William B. Addison,** President of Maxivia LLC, assistant professor of criminal justice, martial arts instructor, and former police officer and trainer for a SWAT and emergency response team

"I really didn't want to have my knee replaced because of the time it would take away from my work and because I was told I wouldn't ever be able to kneel normally again. Prolotherapy was my best chance to avoid surgery so I took it and I am glad I did."
—**Herb Butscher,** data processing manager

"I wouldn't be walking without Dr. Shiple."
—**Charlotte D. Kidd, M. Ed.,** independent writer, professional gardener, garden coach, horticulture educator, www.inthegardendesign.us

"I always tell everyone about prolotherapy. I'd like to do a sales pitch to college athletic departments about RIT because it is so much better than surgery. I would go to Dr. Shiple for anything that happened to me."

    —**Matthew Atkinson**, Penncrest High School and Lycoming College football player

"Dr. Shiple is a very capable, confident, relaxed sort of a guy. He doesn't act like he knows it all, even though he might. I know he's a foremost authority—and getting to be the foremost authority—and that gives me confidence in him. He's so far ahead of these other guys that it's not even funny. He's on the edge of what's happening, what's new, and what's working."

    —**Michelle McKinney**, executive secretary/administrative assistant

"Dr. Shiple is an innovative, forward thinker with cutting-edge technology. What has really helped is his bedside manner, which is the best of any doctor I have ever gone to. He really cares. He has a true relationship with his patients."

    —**Karla K. Atkins**, homemaker

REGENERATIVE HEALING FOR LIFE

A NEW PARADIGM TO TREAT INJURIES AND PAIN WITHOUT SURGERY

BRIAN J. SHIPLE, D.O.
& MARLISE WIND, M.S.

JocDoc Press
Springfield, Pennsylvania

The stories in the book are true; individual names and identifying characteristics of the individuals in the stories have been changed to protect their privacy.

Every effort has been made to ensure the information contained in this book is complete and accurate. However, because of the rapidly evolving nature of regenerative healing, the authors, publishers, and all other persons and entities associated with this book cannot guarantee the accuracy of all information contained herein. The ideas, procedures, and suggestions contained in this book are not intended as a substitute for consulting with your physician. All matters regarding your health require careful, thoughtful, individual medical supervision. The authors, the publishers or any other person or entity associated with them or with this book or mentioned herein shall not be liable or responsible for any loss or damage allegedly arising from any information, case studies, therapies, recommendations, suggestions, etc in this book or from information readers obtain from websites, articles, books, organizations, physicians, or other medical practitioners mentioned in this book.

At the time of writing there are no formal residencies available in regenerative injection techniques, interventional orthopedics, or integrative orthopedic medicine. Hence any physician licensed as a medical or osteopathic doctor can legally perform these procedures. The authors strongly recommend that doctors only perform these procedures after sufficient education, training, and experience. No person associated with this book is responsible if a reader seeks help from an insufficiently trained physician.

Patients desiring any of the treatments described in this book should carefully consider seeking out the recommendations of the organizations cited, which have a long track record of doing research and training in these fields.

JocDoc Press
c/o The Center for Sports Medicine
905 West Sproul Road, Suite 106
Springfield, PA 19064
(484) 472-8812
orders@regen4life.com

978-0-9858443-0-1 (hardcover)
978-0-9858443-1-8 (paperback)
978-0-9858443-2-5 (ebook)

1. Sports medicine 2. Health and fitness 3. Running 4. Knee pain 5. Shoulder pain 6. Elbow pain 7. Arthritis 8. Headaches 9. Back pain 10. Integrative medicine 11. Alternative medicine 12. Chronic pain

To my brother, Lt. Mark E. Shiple, USN call sign "Gator,"
memorialized at Arlington National Cemetery 1984:
May you still fly on wings of eagles

To Eileen, my beautiful, loving wife, and our daughters Kelly,
Bridget, and Clare, thank you all for your tireless love, support,
and especially, patience
—B.J.S.

To Thomas, my loved and loving husband,
and our beloved daughter, Kyla
—M.W.

CONTENTS

INTRODUCTION

*R*egenerative Healing: A New Paradigm for Treating In-juries and Pain Without Surgery* will introduce you to some amazing, pioneering medical treatments that can profoundly change your outcome if you are injured or suffer from chronic pain. These life-changing treatments have already been used by over one million individuals, but remain virtual-ly unknown to the majority of patients and rarely used by most physicians. These techniques rely on the patient's own physical healing powers to create a bridge between conservative stan-dard of care treatments for musculoskeletal injuries, including headaches, arthritis, and surgery. They are non-invasive, espe-cially compared to surgery. They are relatively inexpensive. Par-adoxically, they are often not covered by insurance, even though the medical system could save billions of dollars with their use.

These life-changing treatments have already been used by over one million individuals, but remain virtually unknown to the majority of patients and rarely used by most physicians.

Integrative orthopedic and interventional orthopedic med-icine methods, including regenerative injection treatments (RIT), are the foundations of this new paradigm. Together, they can help acute and chronic tendon, ligament, and cartilage injuries—torn meniscus, plantar faciosis, carpal tunnel syndrome, and tennis elbow among others—as well as lessen or alleviate arthritic joint pain. There is even a growing body of evidence that the arthritic process can be halted or reversed.

C. Everett Koop, M.D., former Surgeon General of the United States, was both a proponent and a beneficiary of these treatments.[1] So are many elite and professional athletes. Two of the key Pittsburgh Steelers 2009 Super Bowl champion players—Hines Ward and Troy Polamalu—who would not have been able to play without these techniques are also enthusiastic.[2] So are legions of my patients, some of whom have related their stories for this book. *Regenerative Healing for Life* will bring vital information about integrative orthopedics and RIT to the tens of millions of people who suffer from arthritis, other disabling illnesses, and musculoskeletal injuries. It will educate patients about many better alternatives to the treatments and drugs currently used. The new paradigm described in this book can dramatically change how both orthopedic surgery and sports medicine are practiced.

One in four Americans is diagnosed yearly with some kind of musculoskeletal condition that requires medical treatment.[3] Currently, over twenty million people in the United States have osteoarthritis, and this number is rising dramatically.[4] The most recent estimate for the yearly total cost (direct and indirect) for bone and joint problems is $849 billion, or 7.7 percent of the gross domestic product.[5] These costs, to the individual and society alike, will increase with the obesity epidemic, with increased recreational activity among baby boomers and with seniors who are living longer.

The common conservative treatments for musculoskeletal

injuries and illnesses include medication, physical therapy, activity modification, bracing, and steroid and viscosupplement injections. If all these fail, medication to manage pain and surgery are the remaining options. Of the over 500,000 knees and over 250,000 hips replaced each year in the United States, 90 percent of these are surgically successful.[6] But, in up to one-third of the cases, patients are not completely satisfied with their outcome.[7] These surgeries also leave patients with the specter of having to endure revision surgery in ten to twenty years, which is often much less effective.

Almost half of people with musculoskeletal problems have injuries that affect tendons and ligaments. Until the advent of RIT, these patients had few alternatives. While surgery can repair some torn or weakened tendons or ligaments, it can also set the stage for, or exacerbate arthritis.

I am a sports medicine physician specializing in integrative and interventional orthopedics, and in RIT. Eschewing the fast track conventional academic and career track I was on, I began my own practice. In the last decade, I have treated well over 10,000 people with these methods. Like all treatments, these methods have a variable success rate, but I am a passionate advocate for them. I have a personal as well as professional understanding of how they fill a critical gap in treatment. I have had an approximately 90 percent success rate with every condition I have treated with the new paradigm, except severe arthritis. Even with the latter, I estimate that joint replacement can be avoided or delayed in at least 50 percent of those treated.

Marlise Wind, M.S.—a successful author who has studied and written about health, spirituality, and integrative medicine for over forty years—can vouch for that estimate. She first saw me for arthritic ankle problems caused by repeated severe sprains. The only treatment offered by traditional medicine at that time was ankle fusion. Now, almost a decade after completing her RIT ankle treatments, she has a more stable ankle function than when she first injured her ankle on a college skiing trip. I subsequently treated her moderately arthritic right knee, and using RIT treatments, have delayed a replacement of her severely arthritic left knee for over seven years.

At the time of writing, RIT comprises four types of treatments. Prolotherapy has been used since the 1930s. It consists of a series of injections of lidocaine and dextrose or another proliferant solution. These injections cause inflammation and

> ## Most patients can see and feel a positive difference within a week or two, and sometimes as soon as a day or two, after the injections.

a release of growth factors which trigger the body's immune system to begin the healing cascade that can bring the patient's body back to a condition it enjoyed in the past. Most patients can see and feel a positive difference within a week or two, and sometimes as soon as a day or two, after the injections. Usually prolotherapy only requires a few days of down time, and a week away from sports or training.

The second treatment is platelet-rich plasma treatment (PRP). This form of RIT is the one most widely used now by top athletes and the one that has been covered in the *New York*

Times, USA Today, The Philadelphia Inquirer, and other publications. With PRP, platelets from the patient's own blood are separated and concentrated and then injected into the target area using ultrasound or other radiological guidance to ensure accurate delivery of the PRP. Platelets contain many growth factors that signal stem cells to promote cartilage and soft tissue repair, and positively affect inflammation, bone grafting, wound healing, and blood loss. PRP also possesses antibacterial and antifungal properties. The solution actually contains stem cells, which stimulate growth of new tendon, ligament, bone, meniscus, nerve, and surface cartilage. This treatment can require three to seven days of down time, and up to six weeks away from rigorous training, although some elite athletes have reported speeding up this process.

The third treatment, adult autologous stem cell injection treatment (ASCI), utilizes the patient's bone marrow—a rich source of stem cells—which is harvested, centrifuged, and injected into the injured or degenerated areas. This method, still in its infancy, promises to be particularly advantageous in treating advanced arthritis and severely degenerated tendons and ligaments, as well as chronic fractures.

The fourth and newest treatment is perineural superficial injection treatment (PSI). This treatment generally consists of superficial injections of low dose dextrose and lidocaine. It is the least invasive of the RIT treatments. PSI has thus far proven extremely effective in treating pain caused by irritated or entrapped nerves, and in treating Achilles tendonitis.[8]

RIT not only bridges a critical gap in conventional treatment; it also offers relief to people suffering from conditions that previously had little chance for a cure. When it is taught and practiced with ethical integrity, RIT can prove to be a major tool in the arsenal of treatments for musculoskeletal injuries, for headaches caused by muscle tension, for pinched nerves, for spinal or jaw problems, and for arthritis. Why use of this amazing treatment is not already more widespread and why insurance doesn't yet pay for it—making it "potentially," not yet actually, less expensive for the patient—is a fascinating story upon which I will touch.

Regenerative Healing for Life is your guide to be sure you are getting outstanding care at every stage of injury healing. To fully understand regenerative healing you need to know about what happens when you are injured, both within your body, and within the medical system. You need to comprehend the differences in

---

Regenerative Healing for Life is your guide to be sure you are getting outstanding care at every stage of injury healing.

---

philosophy and treatment of the current and new paradigms. To get the best care for yourself and those you love, you must approach your treatment as an educated consumer. In this book, I will tell you what can happen in your body when you are injured. I will explain how the current paradigm in the medical system treats the injured patient. I will discuss very helpful treatments known to most doctors, but which are not used with frequency. I will lay out the foundation of the philosophy and treatments of the new paradigm. From there, I will explore with you all of the amazing regenerative injection treatments available at this time. Throughout the book, I will be telling you stories of some of the people these treatments have helped.

I will tell you about the history, development, and anatomical workings of all four methods of RIT, and the pros and cons for each of them. You will learn how injuries or illnesses can be treated by each, and what a treatment is actually like. I will describe the ways in which doctors are trained to perform RIT, the countries in which it is being practiced, and the incredible research being done to find new and better ways to use these treatments. I will advise how you can best prepare for a treatment, and what generally happens after. I will tell you how insurance companies decide what they will or won't cover, and how a new drug or medical procedure journeys from research and development to becoming part of the standard of care for a disease state. You will also find out how consumers can affect this process. This book will help you become a more knowledgeable participant in your own healing and continuing care.

I feel a great urgency to get this book into the hands of the millions of people who, every day, suffer from injuries, chronic pain, and degenerative diseases that can be either alleviated or ameliorated. I also realize the critical importance of *Regenerative Healing for Life* being read by physicians. Open-minded doctors need to learn why and how to provide such therapies to the educated consumers who will be seeking them in ever-increasing numbers.

WHAT CAN RIT TREAT?

Following is a list of injuries and illnesses physicians working with integrative orthopedics and regenerative injection treatments have treated successfully up to the time of this writing.

SHOULDER AND ARM PAIN

- Rotator cuff tendonitis, tendinopathy, or partial and full-thickness tears
- Acromio-clavicular joint pain, injury or arthritis
- Bicipital tendinosis and tears
- Cartilage tears, including labral and chondral surface cartilage tears
- Shoulder and elbow arthritis
- Joint instability chronic subluxation
- Impingement
- Frozen shoulder
- Medial and lateral epicondylitis (golfer's and tennis elbow)
- Ulnar/radial collateral ligament sprain or tear
- Radial/ulnar/median nerve entrapment

BACK PAIN

- Sacroiliac joint arthritis/ instability
- Facet joint arthritis/instability
- Cluneal nerve/spinal nerve entrapment
- Spinal nerve inflammation and injury
- Disc herniation or tear
- Spinal ligament sprain

HIP, PELVIS, AND THIGH PAIN

- Arthritis
- Cartilage tears/labral tears/ chondral surface tears
- Muscle and tendon injuries around the hip
- Hip girdle muscle pain or injury
- Piriformis syndrome
- Greater trochanteric bursitis/ chronic hamstring tendon problems
- Ischial bursitis
- Groin pain/sports hernia/groin strains/nerve entrapment
- Hamstring tendonitis or tears
- Avascular necrosis of the hip from numerous causes

KNEE PAIN

- Patellar tendinosis and tears
- Quadriceps muscle and tendon injuries
- Ligament sprains/tears
- Joint instability
- Cartilage tears, including meniscus and chondral surface cartilage tears
- Arthritis
- Partial ACL tears

LOWER LEG AND FOOT PAIN

- Plantar fasciosis
- Shin splints/mild chronic exertional compartment syndrome
- Ankle/foot tendinosis and tears
- Ankle/high ankle sprains
- Arthritis of the foot and ankle
- Achilles tendinosis/partial and full-thickness tears
- Foot and leg nerve entrapments, such as tarsal tunnel syndrome
- Morton's neuroma
- Avascular necrosis of the foot/ ankle bones

GENERAL PAIN

- Nerve pain
- Chronic pain
- Chronic regional pain syndrome, type 1
- After surgery pain

These methods are evolving quickly. To learn about new uses for RIT, log on to Regen4Life.com.

CHAPTER ONE
REGENERATION IS POSSIBLE

Miracles happen every day that defy medical explanation. The human body is amazing, both in its ability to perform the many functions essential for life and in its ability to heal itself. Ask any physician and he can likely tell you at least one story of a cure that surprised him. Modern medicine is miraculous in its ability to cure ailments that would have caused total disability or death just a decade ago. While medical school, internship, residency, and fellowship training are all geared to make doctors proactive, one of the primary functions of a really good doctor is to know when to act and when to wait. Experience teaches the benefit of waiting to see whether the body can heal itself.

Regenerative therapies rely on the body's ability to self-heal. Doctors practicing these treatments consider body mechanics and frequently see patients' bodies regenerate some joint, tendon, and ligament functions without surgical intervention. These new-paradigm doctors know that while surgery may help one area, it often doesn't take into account the effect on the rest of the patient's body. Medical attitudes and practices change. An interesting example of this can be found in the current prescribed use of non-steroidal anti-inflammatory drugs (NSAIDs). Once thought to be first line treatment for injuries of most kinds, doctors today are realizing they can interfere with the healing process. Only a few years ago, anyone with a fracture would have been given NSAIDs to control the pain and wean the patient off stronger pain medication. Today, orthopedic surgeons tell their patients with fractures to avoid NSAIDs because they hamper the body's natural ability to heal by inhibiting prostaglandin production, thus keeping fractures from mending well. Just as the use of NSAIDs is being reconsidered, I believe mainstream medicine will soon start rethinking surgery as the usual eventual solution for most unresolved musculoskeletal problems.

This chapter will introduce you to possibilities of regenerative healing through the stories of some of my patients. The chronicles here and those of other patients later in the book will show you how regenerative healing has worked for some people, and how it might work for you.

PROLOTHERAPY FOR ARTHRITIS OF THE KNEE

Eric had run a small handyman business for half of his sixty years. He also did a lot of remodeling in his own home. When I first saw him, he recounted how, one day, he carried an air conditioner up a flight of steps, resting it on his right knee in between the steps. This caused him a great deal of pain. He went to see an orthopedic surgeon who told him he had arthritis in his right knee and would need a knee replacement in a few years. The orthopedic surgeon followed the correct conservative course of treatments, giving him cortisone shots and a brace for support, as well as sending him to physical therapy to strengthen the muscles around his knee. Eric followed this course of treatment for the better part of a year. During this time, he also noticed that his left kneecap made a clicking sound which his doctor said was also from arthritis.

His friend, who had been my patient, encouraged Eric to see

me. Because Eric had completed the proper conservative course of treatment, I went right to prolotherapy with him. He had six injections in the joint of his right knee spread over about nine months. He reported that he had no pain after the injections and was able to immediately return to work. Eric reported feeling that his right knee was stable after the six injections, but he wanted me to work on his left knee because he had been over-working it while his right knee healed. After six injections in his left knee, he reported that it was also feeling stable. He continues with maintenance injections on both knees approximately once a year. He wore the brace on his right knee for years after I initially treated him, but then no longer felt the need for it. Four years after completing treatment on both knees, Eric reported that he no longer experienced pain in either.

PROLOTHERAPY FOR PLANTAR FASCIOSIS

A number of years after I saw Eric, his wife Joanne developed pain every time she put weight on her left foot. When I initially interviewed her, she told me one of her favorite leisure activities was walking on the beach. However, the foot pain had become so severe she could barely walk to the bathroom.

"I had to tip-toe on the foot that hurt, and I couldn't walk barefoot at the beach at all. It got so that I avoided going to the beach." She went to her podiatrist who diagnosed her as having plantar faciosis, an inflammation of the thick, tendon-like ligament on the bottom of the foot which connects the heel bone to the toes, thus helping maintain the arch of the foot. Since she had been going to him for over twenty years for a variety of minor foot problems, she trusted whatever he told her. The first process he suggested was wrapping her foot. She would go to him every week to have it wrapped with tape. It did not help. Then he ordered a flexible boot that kept the foot in an upright position during sleep. She wore it every night for months. She reported that it helped when she was lying down, but it did not help her when she was walking.

"Finally he told me there was nothing else he could do for me except send me for surgery. I didn't want to have that done in the summer, be in a cast and ruin our vacation plans. So I just put up with the pain." At Eric's urging, after almost a year of suffering, she came to see me.

When Joanne came to me, she had completed the conservative course of care for plantar faciosis. Her remaining options were surgery, prolotherapy, or experimental treatments. The

---

"I could not believe the relief I had. I felt as if I was in heaven. The pain came back a little gradually, but after the second shot, I didn't have any more pain until a month later, close to my next visit."

---

only reason I jumped right to regenerative healing is that she had gone through everything reasonable with another doctor and did not get better with this conservative care approach. I didn't need to repeat it. So, I treated her right away with prolotherapy and, to her amazement, after the first shot she said the pain was 90 percent better.

"I could not believe the relief I had. I felt as if I was in heaven. The pain came back a little gradually, but after the second shot,

I didn't have any more pain until a month later, close to my next visit. Four shots were all I needed," Joanne reported. I told her to come back if the pain returned, but many years later, she is still pain free. Neither Eric nor Joanne reported experiencing much pain after their treatments. Each of them only had a little bit of swelling and neither even needed to take acetaminophen. Joanne's advice to potential patients is, "Go as soon as you have a problem. Don't wait as long as I did."

PROLOTHERAPY FOR BACK INJURIES

Simon, an Englishman who settled in the suburban Philadelphia area, loves gardening. He takes care of his own large suburban garden and teaches horticulture at several locations. I first took care of him using conventional sports medicine for back problems. Later, he returned with additional back problems that were keeping him from doing the gardening he loved. Following my protocol of first trying conservative treatments, I sent him to physical therapy, and then tried steroid injections since he had two large herniations. None of this provided relief, and Simon was still in too much pain to get back to work. Having exhausted more conservative treatment, I suggested prolotherapy. Simon agreed.

The first time I treated him, I treated his whole lower back, since this would give him the most stability. Simon expressed concern he might have to be immobilized for a couple of days after his treatment. To his surprise, he wasn't hurting when he left the office, and the next morning, his back felt okay. Since the pain he expected never materialized, he thought that was great. The next time he came in for an appointment, he was anxious about what I would find, but I could not find any problem areas that I had to treat. That one treatment was the end of his debilitating back problems, and on a magnetic resonance imaging (MRI) scan he had six months after, it showed that one of the herniations was completely healed, and the other had greatly improved. Simon has had minor problems since, but they have easily resolved with "tune-up treatments."

Simon also had prolotherapy close to a dozen times to treat severe tennis elbow. He reported that he needed to keep his arm in a sling for three or four days after each session, but that the tennis elbow resolved at the end of treatment. He also had arthritis beginning in his shoulder where it connects with the collarbone. After three prolotherapy treatments, he reported the arthritis issue had resolved. Since beginning prolotherapy treatments, Simon has been able to go back to gardening, and continues helping to make his town a more beautiful place.

Now, Simon tells me, "I am a perpetual motion machine. I would recommend that people go online, find out about prolotherapy and consider it. I feel a lot better because of the treatments I've had."

RIT FOR SCIATIC PAIN

Leon is in his early thirties and works for a major company supporting the sales staff. While he does some traveling, he spends the majority of his time in the office. In his free time, Leon was an outdoor runner who averaged thirty to forty miles a week. One day he was on a long run when, at about the eleventh mile, he felt a sensation of fire running up his leg. He told me he walked back home and took a few days off from running.

"At that point," said Leon, "it was too little, too late." Leon went to see an orthopedic surgeon. Over the next year, he went to six other highly reputed orthopedic surgeons. He described himself as being in non-stop pain that would begin in his lower back, run all the way past his knee and into his ankle. He was given a variety of medications to dull the pain but found that the medicines bothered his stomach. He went through four different rounds of physical therapy.

"After three or four appointments with each doctor I felt like it was just another wild goose chase," Leon told me. "I was told every time that they were not sure what was going on, so they would send me for more tests. Meanwhile, I was trying to figure out how I was going to continue working and commuting to my job. Because of the pain, I had difficulty sitting and had to get out of the car every fifteen minutes to stretch. I tried sitting on pillows. I cut out a square of egg crate foam. I tried towels. You name it, I tried it. Nothing worked.

"Looking back, if I had done core exercises, I would not have locked my hip. I would not have shortened my hamstring, which caused me to run poorly on one side, further damaging my hamstring tendons. I drove my own injury by not balancing out my workouts and ended up with very severe sciatic pain."

When Leon first saw me, he was considering acupuncture; and while I told him I knew of some people who had gotten relief from it, I believed I could offer more effective means to help his condition. I first recommended Leon try myofascial release muscle manipulation, a form of massage that frees up the tissue surrounding a nerve. When Leon came to me, he'd had a lot of treatments, but he had not had good myofascial work. With the kind of injury he had, I wanted him to exhaust conservative options first. His injury was over a very large area, difficult to treat with one RIT treatment. For such an extensive injury I have to ask the patient to come back two times in order to treat the entire area once. I recommended Leon do the myofascial work, to see whether releasing some areas of muscle tension would reduce his injured area. That's what happened. He ended up getting relief in some areas and had his first pain-free day in a year. Unfortunately, the relief didn't last.

Because of the nature of his injury, I then recommended trying PRP rather than prolo. Leon was ready to try anything to relieve the pain. The PRP procedure was long and painful. When Leon left that day, he told me he was sure he would never do it again.

"After the swelling went down," Leon said at our next meeting, "I experienced an immediate drop in pain. I changed my mind about PRP pretty fast. When I got to the six-week mark . . . and I had been sitting on foam at the kitchen table and on top of the couch . . . all of a sudden I realized I could sit on a normal chair and not trigger all the pain. It was then that I realized what an impact PRP was having."

"I went from living a full year in the worst pain imaginable to having my life back."

After several more treatments, he was able to complete his commute without being forced to stop because of pain. After five treatments, he reported feeling 95 percent better. While we both wanted to get him completely better so he could do anything he wanted in terms of running, he reported being happy with what we had achieved. "I went from living a full year in the worst pain imaginable to having my life back," he told me.

RIT FOR HEADACHES

Tiffany was a patient whom I began seeing for headaches when she was in her early twenties. The classic prolotherapy protocol, which works on the ligaments, tendons, and joints in the neck and base of the skull, has helped many of my patients over the years. I have found in some patients that this method is enhanced if I do it right after the patient has had chiropractic or osteopathic manipulation. When manipulation alone and prolotherapy alone did not sufficiently help Tiffany, I tried the manipulation and prolotherapy model. After the first treatment, she had almost a month free of headaches. After six treatments, Tiffany was headache free for years. When she was in her thirties, with several small children, her headaches began to return. At this point I used a different type of regenerative treatment on Tiffany—perineural superficial injections (PSI). In this treatment, the solution I inject, usually very dilute dextrose mixed with a small amount of lidocaine, goes only down to the superficial nerves under the skin, not into the tendons or ligaments.

I had already used PSI on a number of patients, including Susan, who had suffered from chronic migraines for thirty years. Susan's pain was so great that a bad headache could keep her out of work for a week. She even had an occipital nerve stimulator surgically implanted without any release from pain. After Susan's first perineural superficial injections, she had five pain-free days for the first time in thirty years. With each treatment, the pain-free time increased.

To be very clear, there are two major categories of headaches: ones that come from musculoskeletal causes, such as abnormal muscle tension alone or with impact on the nerves in the shoulders, neck, and head. RIT therapies have a very positive record in treating this type of headache. The other type of headache comes from vascular disturbances. I have not had much success over the years treating these.

Because of my experiences with Tiffany, Susan, and many other patients, I am optimistic about how both classic prolotherapy and perineural superficial injections can help people who suffer from chronic tension headaches and musculoskeletally induced migraine headaches.

PROLOTHERAPY FOR TMJ

Maryann, a thirty-year-old stay-at-home mother of three children, comes from a small town. She suffered with chronic pain stemming from hamstring and elbow injuries, and temporomandibular joint (TMJ) dysfunction. Rather than being supportive, her husband was verbally abusive, accusing her of faking pain. She came to me, and, given the extent and locations of her injuries, I immediately suggested working with prolotherapy. After each treatment her chronic pain subsided, and she gained confidence and strength. She eventually found the courage to stand up to her husband. She began to get more physically active and joined a hiking club. Over time, she shared with them details of her home situation. They helped her to find the fortitude to leave her husband and start a new life with her children. Very happy now, she attributes her improvement in life to the prolotherapy treatments that allowed her to conquer her chronic pain.

RIT FOR ACL TEARS

Yolanda was a strong but quiet woman training for her black belt in karate. While sparring, she injured her knee. If she tried to lean on that knee to do a kick, the knee would collapse, and she would fall down on the mat. She went to several orthopedic surgeons, and they told her she had a partial anterior cruciate ligament (ACL) tear in her knee and therefore didn't need surgery yet. She took about a year looking at her alternatives to surgery and, as she was researching, came across my name. She came to me and said, "I can't go on this way." Upon examination, I found that enough fibers of the ACL were still there to give her a chance of healing through prolotherapy. After four treatments, her knee was solid, and, when I repeated her MRI, it was completely normal.

Prolotherapy works well with ligaments in the knee, the shoulder, the elbow, and the hand, which means it's useful in treating carpal tunnel syndrome, tennis elbow, and golfer's elbow.

I presented her case at a regional meeting at a Philadelphia hospital for a group of orthopedic surgeons, therapists, and trainers, where I'd been asked to speak about prolotherapy's potential use in sports medicine. With her permission, I displayed Yolanda's before and after MRIs and showed where I placed the needle.

The MRI picture looked impressive, like the ACL was almost completely torn. But Yolanda still had a ligament, and her MRI confirmed it was partially intact, although hanging on by a thread. I inserted the needle into the footprint of where the

ACL is supposed to be. We did four treatments a month apart, and then I ordered another MRI. Her knee looked like she had a brand-new ACL. It looked like it was never injured to begin with. You could hear a pin drop when I presented the case to the audience. Yolanda went on to complete her black belt and to compete at a very high level in her sport.

I've had several traditional sports medicine docs say to me, "You know, we have a prolotherapist in our community who says he can rebuild a completely torn ACL. What do you say to that, Shiple?" My response is that this claim is ridiculous. Prolotherapy can't cure a completely torn ACL. You can't repair something that's not there. When an ACL is completely torn there is nothing left to repair; it has to be reconstructed. While prolotherapy can't cure a complete ACL tear, it can help patients who have partially torn or stretched their ligaments to the point that they are no longer doing their job.

Prolotherapy works well with ligaments in the knee, the shoulder, the elbow, and the hand, which means it's useful in treating carpal tunnel syndrome, tennis elbow, and golfer's elbow, as well as the other disorders I have written about in this chapter. It can also be a very powerful tool in helping heal partially torn ligaments. It can even work with fully torn ligaments that don't blow up and disappear like the ACL does. Ligaments are still there when they are completely torn, but are lying all stretched out. When I do prolotherapy on such ligaments and follow it with proper physical therapy, the ligaments grow thicker and stronger, tighten, and begin to reconnect. Before you know it, the patient has healed to the point he has a normal ligament that I can see with diagnostic ultrasound.

RIT FOR MULTIPLE INJURIES

Michael had been involved in martial arts and self-defense instruction since he was five years old. He had worked as a police officer for almost twenty years. In both his avocation as a martial artist and in his job, he had suffered numerous injuries. Several years ago, while involved in apprehending a suspect, he severely injured his knee.

He had surgery at a prominent orthopedic center for a tear in his meniscal cartilage and was back to his normal activities, both on and off duty, within six weeks. The next year he was involved in another apprehension that turned violent. Again, the same knee was injured.

"It blew up like a balloon," Michael said, "and felt soft." He returned to the orthopedic surgeon who drained it, injected it with cortisone, and prescribed an anti-inflammatory medication and a knee brace. He returned to work using the brace. A few weeks later, he was sent out on a domestic violence call. One of the people involved kicked Michael directly across the knee brace. He returned to the doctor the next day and started going to physical therapy while continuing with his job.

"I'm used to injuries," Michael said when I first saw him, "I'm used to going to doctors and I always fight to get back to 100 percent. However, after this third knee injury I was in so much pain it was horrible. When the physical therapy didn't work and the transcutaneous electrical nerve stimulation (TENS) unit didn't control my pain, the orthopedic surgeon told me about you."

After I took Michael's history and performed a physical examination, I suggested trying prolotherapy since he had already exhausted the conservative treatment options and had such a severe injury. This provided Michael with the first relief he'd had since the second knee injury. Michael felt it gave him another chance to be fully functioning in life. He continued working even though he would sometimes need to stop his patrol car and move his leg so that it wouldn't freeze up. It turned out that the force of the kick he'd received across the brace had caused permanent damage to Michael's saphenous nerve. Surgeons told him the nerve was so badly damaged there was nothing they could do. They had no treatment to get this nerve to come back. Like having a spinal cord injury that would paralyze you for the rest of your life, that nerve was not supposed to regenerate. I talked to a colleague and asked him whether he had any experience with using PRP on damaged nerves and getting them to come back. I knew there were a number of doctors doing autologous stem cell injections (ASCI) on spinal cord injuries and seeing some patients recover partial functionality if the injury wasn't too old. Since this was before I was trained in ASCI, I asked this colleague about doing PRP instead. He said he knew of physicians who had gotten decent results from using PRP.

I said to my colleague, "What the hell, this guy has nothing else to lose. He is not a surgical candidate, so he is looking at permanent pain for the rest of his life. If he agrees, I'm going to try it." Prior to treating Michael's nerve, I sent him to two top-notch Philadelphia neurosurgeons who specialized in peripheral nerve injuries. They told him they could not offer him any treatment other than nerve ablation, which means to kill the nerve. This was not offered with a significant chance of success, so Michael refused this as his only chance at controlling his pain.

With Michael's consent, I treated him with PRP hydrodissection along the injured nerve to see if it would help the nerve repair itself. We did three treatments for Michael, and he got about 75 percent better. It then took about two months to recover from his fourth treatment, but after that time he felt about 85 to 90 percent better. He no longer has numbness in his foot, unless he twists his knee or foot in a way that stretches the nerve. Then he'll get a zing, but it goes away as quickly as it comes. His pain is under very good control now; not perfect, but good control. He knows how to be careful and really has adapted. He is running, biking, walking, playing with his kids—all things he couldn't do before treatment. He is also working out like a fiend, and, since he was unable to work out before, that makes him really happy. Michael had a complicated medical problem but an intense drive to function as normally as possible. He is doing unbelievably well. He said that if he never got any better than this, he would still be very happy with the results he has obtained.

"I believe PRP and prolo have gotten me where I am today. I'm swimming and running. I can play with, and hold my children. All the other doctors told me I would never be able to do those things again. Do I have an injury and pain? Absolutely, but it is manageable because of PRP and prolo. Medication helps to a certain degree but, unlike medication, prolo and PRP aren't masking agents. They are a rehabilitation process."

When Michael last came in to see me, he announced that he was even better, so good that he was leaving to climb Mount Kilimanjaro the following week, and that he had just finished running a marathon. While teaching and pursuing his Ph.D., he also manages to work out for three hours a day.

Maybe you have seen parts of yourself or someone you care about reflected in one of the patients I've introduced to you in this chapter. You'll hear more details about some of these patients and meet many others in the chapters that follow. These patients amazed me in their ability to heal from injuries and ill-nesses that could have condemned them to a life of pain and/or disability. Their courage and tenacity has taught me that, with the proper treatment, regenerative healing is indeed possible.

CHAPTER TWO
MY JOURNEY TO REGENERATIVE HEALING

After five years of practicing sports medicine, I found myself in a condition similar to that of some my patients described in the last chapter. I was getting ready to turn in my disability insurance papers. It was becoming increasingly difficult for me to work as a doctor who needed physical strength to examine and manipulate my patients' injured limbs. Being weak because of chronic pain was an unusual and unpleasant experience for me. Up to this point in my life, I had been blessed with strength, agility, and good health. My current disability was the result of an automobile accident that exacerbated injuries I had sustained as a high school football player. Being injured, in pain, and considering disability were definitely not part of my life plan, although my situation certainly made me empathize with many patients I saw in similar situations.

Prior to this time, I was on a high-powered career track that led me to direct one of the top sports medicine fellowship programs in the country. Hired right out of my fellowship at Penn State University, I became an assistant director of the Crozer-Keystone Family Practice Residency Program in Springfield, Pennsylvania, a suburb of Philadelphia. Quickly I was named Director and Division Chief of Sports Medicine at the hospital, then Director of the Sports Medicine Fellowship Program.

Because of medical school loans and having three daughters in private school, I was also working some nights as an emergency medicine attending physician in Newark, Delaware. My weekends were often as full of career-oriented activities as my weeks. I acted as chief medical officer for the Keystone State Games, the Pennsylvania Senior Games, and the Philadelphia Triathlon. I was active giving numerous local and national presentations on a wide variety of topics, including on-field management of the injured athlete, triage of school injuries and medical emergencies, exercise-induced asthma, how to start an exercise program, osteopathic manipulation therapy, and joint and soft tissue injection techniques.

In confronting my frustration at not being able to help patients more, I began a journey to look for something else to offer.

In addition, I was working at a number of schools as a team physician for football, wrestling, and ice hockey. I was a volunteer team physician for the U.S. Olympic Committee Training Center and a liaison team physician for the San Francisco Giants Baseball Team when they played in Philadelphia. I was the founding medical director of the Philadelphia Triathlon at Fairmount Park, and served in the post for two years, overseeing an athlete population of over 1,500 and a spectator population of several thousand more. I was a team physician for the one hundredth running of the Boston Marathon, and in my sparse free time, I enjoyed being with my wife and daughters, playing golf, snow skiing, scuba diving, and bicycling.

To outward appearances, I was a quintessentially successful sports medicine doctor, but inwardly I harbored some doubts about my profession's limitations. By the time my physical problems forced me to consider disability I had already reached the conclusion that while I could accurately diagnose most patients' problems, I could only help a certain percentage of them. After trying anti-inflammatory medications, physical therapy, osteopathic manipulation, braces, orthotics, steroid or viscosupplement injections, I felt I didn't really have much else to offer them. I knew eventually they would end up seeing a surgeon who would either do surgery or not. If they weren't offered surgery, many times it meant a life of further pain, muscular or joint degeneration, and disability. While I know surgery has a definite place in treating musculoskeletal problems, I would often see patients who had undergone surgery and were not satisfied with their results.

FINDING PROLOTHERAPY

In confronting my frustration at not being able to help patients more, I began a journey to look for something else to offer. It led to my exploring acupuncture, myofascial manipulation, and trigger point therapy, and also being trained in some of these methods. While I observed these techniques were good for treating a percentage of symptoms and issues, I concluded even they were not really getting to the root cause of the problem. That often lies in tendons and ligaments, which have become diseased, torn or lax from injury, age, or overuse.

At a conference I attended, I saw there was a lecture to be given by a doctor who was a prolotherapist. I knew little about this treatment, and was curious. The scheduled speaker, also a team physician, had to make a last-minute trip with Lance Armstrong and his cycling team. The substitute speaker who came in was an expert at prolotherapy, but not at public speaking. When he started there were about 300 doctors in the room, and all of us were glued to our seats. We had just finished listening to a great presentation by Brian Halpern, M.D., who had traveled to Vietnam providing medical care for disabled veterans in wheelchair tricycles. They had participated in a big race with both Vietnamese and American veterans going down the Ho Chi Minh trail for thirty days. When he concluded his tale, you could have heard a pin drop. By the end of the prolotherapist's talk, you could have still heard a pin drop—because there were only a handful of us left in the room. Yet, I immediately grasped the importance of his message about prolotherapy and its possibilities. I started looking at this as a potential treatment. I found and read articles on it and talked to some patients who had undergone the treatment.

About a year later, I attended another presentation on prolotherapy given by Shawn Kerger, D.O., who was a trusted friend and expert in the field of sports medicine. He was training in prolotherapy and using it on his athletes. He recounted a particular case of a Division I college running back who'd had a good year as a freshman with about 1,000 yards rushing. Then he injured his ankle and ran only about 300 yards in his sophomore year. He had prolotherapy in the off-season, and when he came back, he had well over 2,000 yards rushing in both his junior and senior years. He went on to become a Heisman candidate, was drafted to play in the NFL, and has been enjoying a very successful career as a running back for over a decade.

When my colleague explained what he did, how he did it, how good this football player's ankle is now, and how well he was able to perform after prolotherapy, I said to myself, "This is it. This is what I've been looking for." The first course I took in prolotherapy was in Maine at the New England College of Osteopathic Medicine. It was given by a group under the umbrella organization of the American Academy of Osteopathy (AAO). The doctors who started that course have since written an excellent textbook on the subject.[1] I spent close to 200 hours in extra training, on my own time, to become knowledgeable about performing prolotherapy procedures. Within the first year of learning how to do prolotherapy, I was invited to teach it since I was already a recognized educator in injection techniques at the national level. It took more than three years for me to learn about prolotherapy, get trained in it, and start performing it on my patients.

At the same time I was on this journey, I was suffering from severe back and shoulder injuries I'd sustained in a car accident. These exacerbated residual high school football injuries. I had severe tennis elbow, rotator cuff disease, and shoulder instability. Together, it all made examining patients, manipulating their limbs, and performing injections a painful experience for me. Just trying to resist a patient's muscle contraction—something I had to do in a thorough physical exam—would make me see stars. After trying to perform osteopathic manipulation on a larger athlete's spine, I remember feeling a burning leg pain shooting down to my toes. Even riding my road bike required getting off every twenty minutes in order to stretch my back and hamstrings. If I went any further, my feet would fall asleep for the rest of the ride. Playing golf at that point was out of the question. The mere act of swinging a club caused left-sided arm, elbow, and shoulder pain so severe I had to decline invitations to golf with friends. I remember once when I was working on a deck I built, I exacerbated my back and sciatic pain to the point where I could hardly move for a solid week.

On the verge of throwing in the towel and filing for disability,

---

I'm a card-carrying member of the prolo club, so I know what you're going to go through.

I decided instead to use myself as a guinea pig. I traveled five hours from Philadelphia to Connecticut to be treated by Paul Tortland, D.O., one of the doctors I had met at the prolothera-py course. Since I was making the long drive, I figured I would get my money's worth. I asked him to treat my lower back, my right knee, my left wrist, left elbow, and left shoulder all on the same day. I had well over a dozen injections. My wife and our infant daughter rode up with me and my wife drove back. I took one tablet of acetaminophen with codeine after the treatment, and that was it. About a week later, I began to experience sig-nificant pain relief and could do more with my injured left arm. That first treatment helped enough that I returned twice more to Connecticut.

Those first few treatments saved my career. Within two treatments, I was greater than 50 percent better. With the third treatment, I was 80 percent better. I did well enough that I didn't need any treatments after that for a while. I went back to the gym and started working out again, and I began riding my bike. I could ride for an hour before my feet would fall asleep. My body felt so good I even tried golf. Eventually, I got back to playing golf and doing all the things I enjoy up to this day. For me, prolotherapy was definitely a practice changer and a career saver. Seeing what it did for me, I began using it to treat my patients. When one would ask, "Well, what's it like to go through this treatment?" I would reply, "I'm a card-carrying member of the prolo club, so I know what you're going to go through." I think it does help when a patient realizes that the treatment their doctor is recommending is one he has undergone himself. From then on, I kept training more and more in prolotherapy, and, later, in other forms of RIT.

TOP DOC WITH NEW IDEAS

While all this was happening, I was also working to expand the Crozer-Keystone Health System's fellowship program in sports medicine. By the time I started doing prolotherapy, I had been working at Crozer for six years. We were doing well. I was the medical director of a United States Olympic Committee Testing and Treating Center at Crozer's sports facility, the Healthplex. We had affiliations with schools and universities. I was speaking at the national level on all different kinds of topics concerning sports medicine. I was chosen one of the top doctors in the Philadelphia area by *Philadelphia Magazine* in 2002, and was chosen as a Crozer's Teaching Attending Physician of the Year eight of the thirteen years I worked there.

The fellowship program I was directing was a straightforward M.D. program. However, the amount of prolotherapy I was doing skewed my practice toward chronic pain injuries. Keep in mind, the medical definition of a chronic injury is any injury that hasn't healed in six weeks. Close to 50 percent of my patients were either being evaluated for, beginning, or completing treatment in prolotherapy. The other 50 percent were receiving more traditional sports medicine treatments. As a physician, I want to treat and help any patient I can. Because I was willing to treat patients with chronic injuries or pain, I was no longer running a traditional M.D. sports medicine fellowship. The sports medicine students who were looking for that kind of acute injury-focused fellowship program would choose another one. The people who came to our program were interested in some of the new treatments I was pursuing. We always got our top picks because we ran a very good program, did our job well, and had a good reputation.

The longer I taught, the more I realized I got greater gratification from treating and healing patients than from teaching fellows. And the job changed. My practice became so packed with patients it took two months before I could even bring a patient back for follow up. It became impossible to properly care for my patients. The company I was working for was resistant to letting me hire anybody else to do this work, so the more patients I had, the longer it took to get in to see me for a new or follow-up appointment. I just couldn't give the kind of care I wanted to give my patients, so I finally made the decision to leave and go out on my own. The move away from teaching and administering a fellowship program really freed me up to explore new ideas and techniques.

SEEKING CUTTING-EDGE CARE

Cutting-edge care was what my patient (and now co-author) Marlise Wind wanted. An author of ten books, one about integrative healing and several about cross-cultural healing techniques and philosophies, she was annoyed to find herself in a situation that only seemed to have a few allopathic options—none of them very appealing.

Marlise had initially injured her left ankle in the 1960s the first time she went skiing. Her college medical center cast her severely injured ankle, gave her aspirin, and told her to stay in bed for a few days. These are all things we would never do for a badly sprained ankle in sports medicine today. When the cast came off a month later, she went back to her normal activities with no further treatment. Physical therapy was much less widely prescribed in those days. For years as a young professional, Marlise said, she ran around New York City in heels. Later, she replaced these with the negative heel shoes then popular, changing her body mechanics and contributing to her spraining her already-injured ankle again and again. Over the years, she tried rest, immediate activity, ice, heat, stretching, exercise, massage of all kinds, acupuncture, herbs, and a lot of aspirin. By the time I saw her, she had sprained that ankle over twenty-five times.

In the 1990s she suffered another injury. After years of misdiagnosis, she was told she had severe trauma-induced osteoarthritis of her right hip. At that time, the orthopedic surgeon told her she was too young to have a hip replacement and to come back when she had to crawl in. Marlise waited five years, until she could barely walk. She reported that her right hip replacement went well, and she'd had minimal problems with her hip since.

Because of how long a time Marlise walked with a severely arthritic right hip, her left ankle and knee took much of the strain of her uneven gait. The orthopedic surgeon told her a single or double knee replacement was in her near future. When her left ankle started to act up again she went back to the orthopedic institute and saw one of the foot and ankle doctors there. He made her a pair of orthotics and discussed the possibility of fusing her ankle, which was, at that point, the most common option for severe ankle arthritis. The orthotics helped her for a period of time but then her ankle really began hurting and she needed a cane in order to walk.

Marlise told me in our initial interview, "Even using a cane, I'm exhausted from the effort of walking." Her psychiatrist husband and several other friends in the medical field told her they had heard about a physician doing treatments with injections that might help her. She limped into my office about two months before she was scheduled to leave on a vacation requiring lots of walking. After taking her history and examining her, I explained what prolotherapy was and how it might help her. I told her she could have two treatments before she left on her trip, and those two might be enough to increase her mobility.

In the first treatment, I gave her over a dozen injections in her ankle joint and in the tendons and ligaments surrounding it. After the treatment, she reported her ankle swelled to the size of a baseball and hurt. When the initial inflammation subsided, she discovered she was relying a lot less on the cane.

Six weeks later, she came back for the second series of injections, and, by the time she went on vacation, she told me she was walking with a slight rather than pronounced limp, and only needed the cane for longer walks or when her ankle was really tired.

When she returned from her trip, she continued the prolotherapy treatments. At the end of the initial six treatments, her ankle felt more stable than it had since she had first injured it. After these, she returned to me as needed for "tune-ups" to keep the arthritis in her ankle under control. Over a decade later she still has very stable ankle function, and infrequent pain.

CHASING HER INJURIES

Since prolotherapy had worked so well on her ankle, she decided to try it on her knees. Her left knee at this point was severely arthritic and her right knee had moderate arthritis. They were both coming along well with prolotherapy treatments until one icy day when a young woman lost control of her car and caused a multi-vehicle accident in which Marlise was involved. Her car was spun 180 degrees and the accident injured her left shoulder, knee, and ankle as well as giving her a nasty concussion and problems with her spine. Because of the success she'd had with prolotherapy, she decided to treat her accident injuries only with me. A year or so after the accident I told her that I wasn't sure she would be able to bounce back from the injuries it had inflicted. But through prolotherapy and, later, other forms of regenerative injection treatment (RIT) she has managed to maintain function, and the ability to keep exercising.

"Sometimes it felt like I was chasing my own injuries," Marlise said. "When I would get my left knee relatively pain free, my right knee would begin to hurt. Later I experienced pain in my big toe, my heel, and my lower back. All of my injuries—except for my severely arthritic knee—have been treated solely with prolotherapy. It has worked every place I've been treated with the exception of my left shoulder injured in the accident. The accident aggravated advanced degenerative arthritis already present in my shoulder and, although I still have it, prolotherapy has kept it under control."

When the prolotherapy was not enough to resolve the arthritis in her left knee, I suggested Marlise try a series of PRP treatments. They gave her a lot more relief, but not the ability to exercise very vigorously. She had bone spurs on the knee and her cartilage was wearing thin. Because we had reached the point where surgery was the next option, I offered to use her as a test subject when I began giving ASCI treatment. We are both pleased with the results and she reports being able to walk and exercise more.

WHY HAVEN'T YOU HEARD ABOUT RIT?

Marlise began to talk with me about writing a book about prolotherapy a few years after I began treating her. When I became established in my own practice, Marlise was ready to begin work. We are both more convinced than ever of the necessity of a book that lets people know there is another healing paradigm for treating injuries and musculoskeletal degeneration.

In the business of medicine in the United States, it costs in the neighborhood of $800 million dollars[2] in testing and marketing to get a new drug or piece of medical equipment approved by the Food and Drug Administration (FDA), covered by insurance, and known to the general public. Since no pharmaceutical or medical device company stands to make back that amount from the drugs or devices now used for regenerative injection treatment (RIT), it is unlikely there will be corporate-sponsored research in this area. Consequently, one of the few ways for it to become an accepted method of treating otherwise untreatable injuries is by informing the general public, via the lay press, of the quality research already conducted and in progress.

Although there have been about 100 research projects published on prolotherapy, most have ranged from well-designed placebo controlled trials without randomization to case-controlled studies, prospective case-series studies, or opinions from respected authorities based on clinical experience.[3] In medical terms, these are Level II and III and IV studies. What is needed for prolotherapy to gain mainstream acceptance are Level I studies, which are sizable properly designed, randomized controlled trials.[4] Again, no corporate entity stands to make millions or billions if prolotherapy becomes covered by Medicare and other insurance providers. Consequently, it is difficult for RIT researchers to find the funding they need to conduct the studies that would make this treatment acceptable to insurers.

Until large, controlled studies show beyond a shadow of a doubt that RIT works better than a placebo, it is unlikely to be covered by the commercial insurance companies. So RIT will remain outside mainstream medicine's "standard of care," and only available to patients from physicians who, like me, seek to treat their patients with any treatment that has a reasonable research record, is safe and works on real people. Once you see the potential efficacy of this option, I trust you will begin to question why RIT is not practiced by more physicians or covered by insurance.

CHAPTER THREE
WHY YOU SHOULD KNOW
ABOUT REGENERATIVE HEALING

If you've never had an injury that required medical care, you are indeed lucky. One in four Americans is diagnosed yearly with some kind of musculoskeletal condition that requires medical treatment.[1] Injuries are the leading cause of death for people in the one-year-old to forty-four-year-old age group, killing more people than cancer, HIV, the flu, and heart disease.[2] In 2010, the last year for which statistics were available at the time of writing, over 180,000 people died from injuries, almost three million people were hospitalized for an injury, and at least thirty million people were treated for non-fatal injuries in U.S. hospital emergency rooms.[3]

How do all of these people get injured? Motor vehicle accidents account for 37 percent of injuries; falls account for 16 percent; and the rest are caused either by self- or other-inflicted violence, or by unclassified incidents.[4] The leading cause of trauma hospital admissions among adolescents and young adults is injury to the lower extremities: broken toes, Achilles tendon injuries, sprained ankles, injured knees, hamstring tears, and so on. Over 235,000 young people are hospitalized for such conditions each year.[5] According to the CDC, yearly an estimated 80,000 Americans sustain traumatic brain injuries (TBI) that result in disability.[6] Over five million Americans live with TBI.

Approximately 11,000 people each year sustain spinal cord injuries (SCI), and there are at least 200,000 Americans living with SCI.[7] Over fifty million people in the United States have some type of arthritis, the most common being osteoarthritis.[8] Arthritis is the nation's most common cause of disability, limiting the activities of twenty-one million Americans.[9]

THE HEALING CASCADE

How you deal with an injury initially has a profound effect on whether and how it will affect you in the future. To get the proper initial care, you must understand what can occur when an injury is treated well, untreated or treated improperly. As long as a patient arms him or herself with sufficient knowledge, I'm in favor of people looking after themselves and not running to the doctor for every small injury. Yet when it comes to self-treatment, all too often the individual is treating the symptoms of the healing process when he believes he is treating the symptoms of the injury!

I'm not the first to observe this, but the human body is a pretty miraculous system. When we first hurt ourselves, so long as our self-healing system is uncompromised by other factors, which I will later discuss, our body does everything it can to heal the injury. It immediately releases prostaglandin (among other chemicals), a powerful and versatile fatty acid that launches an inflammatory cascade. This cascade brings to the injured area white blood cells and platelets, which secrete certain growth factors and proteins that begin the healing process. That is why an injured area swells, feels painful and warm. But this intense healing cascade does not last long. It burns itself out, usually after four to five days, although some of it lingers up to ten days. This initial period is critical. If this phase isn't allowed to progress naturally or for long enough, the latter healing stages won't be as effective.

In the later healing phases, which can last for weeks or months, depending on the severity of the injury, the body stops producing the chemicals we initially needed, and works to develop new collagen and blood vessels that finish the healing process. After about six weeks, initial healing should be completed. If pain remains, it is no longer due to inflammation, but to a chronic injury and joint instability. This is an indication that something prevented ideal healing and the injury would now be classified as chronic, as would the pain. A commonly quoted sta-

---

The human body is amazing in its ability to regenerate if we don't do things to hamper the process.

---

tistic I have read is that if normal phases of the healing process have been allowed to continue unimpeded, then about 85–90 percent of patients will heal from simple injuries without a need for further treatment. We don't yet have a satisfactory answer for the reasons why not everyone fully heals. The combination of genetics and/or medications may exert quite a bit of influence over who heals and who doesn't. Other possible causes are overuse of the injured area during healing, mitigating diseases, inadequate nutrition, and improper care.

Always remember, the human body is amazing in its ability to regenerate if we don't do things to hamper the process.

THE KINETIC CHAIN AND REFLEX INHIBITION

Everybody knows that the foot bone is connected to the ankle, and so forth. I explain to my patients, "We're like an Erector Set that is supposed to move. If one screw is loose, because of a little instability in a ligament or weakness in a tendon, it's going to eventually cause a loosening down the line in the Erector Set, and another screw is going to become loose, and then another one, and another one. . ." This is a simple explanation for the principle behind what is called the kinetic chain. The kinetic chain connects one area of the body to the next through bones, joints, muscles, ligaments, fascia, nerves, lymph, and blood vessels. Kinetic has to do with motion—how we move.

To recover most completely from an injury, you need to understand the principles of how you heal, and what can interfere with the healing process. I will introduce to you important concepts that are unfamiliar to many patients and even to some doctors. However, they have a profound effect on whether, when and how you heal. These terms are reflex inhibition, dynamic stabilization failure, and postural decompensation. Because of the way our bodies are connected, any problem area that goes untreated is likely to have an effect upon other parts of our body. Eventually the whole kinetic chain becomes dysfunctional (this is dynamic stabilization failure), and with dysfunction, there is pain and the possibility of further injury.

Gretchen is an example of this. She came to me on the advice of a friend. Two years before, she had fallen and landed on both knees. She went to her primary doctor and had radiological studies that showed no particular damage, although she was in a lot of pain. She took NSAIDs for a long time to relieve the pain, but it never quite went away. About six months later she began to have pain in her left hip. Again, x-rays showed no specific damage there. A few months later, she began to have pain in her left ankle. It spread to her foot. She went to a number of specialists. Since there was no apparent arthritis, and no measurable nerve damage, she was diagnosed as having fibromyalgia. She tried more medication and some aqua therapy. Her pain continued.

When I looked at Gretchen with diagnostic ultrasound, I found several small ligament and tendon defects in her right knee. Clinically I found evidence of some swollen superficial nerves around her knee, and the ligaments in her left ankle were much looser than they should have been. Gretchen's condition illustrates how one untreated injury can lead to another. The way in which this most often happens is through what is called reflex inhibition, first posited by David C. Reid, M.D.[10] Through his work, and that of Ben Kibler, M.D., I became familiar with the concept in the 1990s.

Reflex inhibition is when the body shuts down certain important muscles around an area that has been injured in an effort to force the individual to rest that damaged part of the body, both preventing exacerbation of the injury and allowing it to heal. In past ages, this likely was an effective way of slowing an injured person down. Today, however, in the age of modern medicine, we can use medications to cover up the pain and allow us to go back to using that part of the body before it is ready. This increases the risk of dynamic stabilization failure, which is what had happened to Gretchen.

All doctors have learned they can mask the discomfort of an injury for a time. However, as long as there's pain, reflex inhibition will be present, at least to some extent, and vice versa. Reflex inhibition goes hand in hand with pain. Both act to prevent further injury like a mother does in keeping a child away from a hot stove. She may bark, "Don't touch that!" and at the same time grab the child's hand, immobilizing the child so he can't hurt himself. This is what reflex inhibition does by shutting down an injured part. By masking the pain, it's possible for the injured individual to override the reflex inhibition.

However, doing so can not only exacerbate the original injury, but also create new injuries. This can happen because reflex inhibition puts the joint in a biomechanical dysfunctional state. The muscles that have been turned off also become overly tight. This causes abnormal joint mechanics and starts to cause increased stress on ligaments about the joint. This causes other muscles to overcompensate to a point and then fail and become weak and tight. Before you know it, dynamic stabilization failure can develop, putting you at risk for further injury down the kinetic chain.

This means that in treatment it is imperative for doctors to consider the injury pattern between all the possible parts of the body that could be injured. Then the doctor needs to either rule them in or out to make an accurate diagnosis of an injury. Consequently, the best treatment plan is to treat the primary pain generator, stop the reflex inhibition, begin to undo the dynamic stabilization failure, and return the regional and distant muscles to normal strength and neuromuscular firing patterns. This takes time, and a deep understanding of the injury progression, the biomechanical stress that injury imparts on the kinetic chain, the healing process, and the individual patient.

Patients seem to fall into one of two categories of healing. Either they heal easily on their own, not developing significant dynamic stabilization failure, or they need to be actively treated in some kind of therapy. This can be at home or with a skilled therapist to retrain their injured muscles to return to a pain-free and functional state. Gretchen fell into the latter category, as most people do. She never received a prescription for the appropriate type of physical therapy at the proper time in her course of treatment. If she had, that might have helped her heal after her initial injury. There are many types of physical therapy, which I will discuss in detail in Chapter Five. Not all are beneficial for all patients at the same stage of injury. Both timing and the skill of the therapist are critical.

One patient I helped through a chronic injury said her doctor called me the "injury whisperer." This drives home an important point: Doctors need to be good listeners to pick up the clues in their patients' stories.

The first step in my treatment of a patient is doing a thorough history and physical in which I really try to listen to his story. Every patient has a story to tell and there I can find the key to his diagnosis. The patient usually gives me the clues in the initial history albeit buried in his story. The physical exam and the diagnostic tests are just confirming what I have already learned from his story. One patient I helped through a chronic injury said her doctor called me the "injury whisperer." We both got a good chuckle out of that label, but it drives home an important aspect of my process. Doctors need to be good listeners to pick up the clues in their patients' stories. This is critical to determine what the original injury was, and whether and how it has affected other parts of the body. Although this would ideally be a routine experience for patients, apparently it isn't.

Luke came to see me and reported, "It hurts for me to grab something off the top of a cabinet." I suspected right away he might have shoulder impingement, stemming from some untreated or poorly treated injury that had led to reflex inhibition. As it turned out when I took his history, Luke had injured his right shoulder about three months earlier, playing racquetball. He had been in pain since then, long enough for many of the fourteen shoulder stabilizing muscles that control shoulder motion to have been automatically turned off in sequence. In order to treat the shoulder, I first needed to figure out what specific injury began the downward spiral and deal with the original pain that started Luke's problem. Only then could I begin to help him reverse the reflex inhibition, and get his shoulder biomechanics back to normal.

When I establish a diagnosis, including any effects of reflex inhibition, the next phase of treatment is determining how to appropriately shut off the patient's pain. If a patient has a swollen arthritic joint, I would examine the area, locating the underlying cause. I would do so using my diagnostic ultrasound equipment, which is capable of providing a much clearer picture of many superficial musculoskeletal problems than an MRI can. I may ask to review an up-to-date x-ray or MRI as well to help see the effects of the injury on the joint and surrounding anatomy. Therapy may be able to help control the pain by using electrical stimulation, ice, heat, or ultrasound. However, a doctor may need to intervene to turn the patient's pain off by using parts of both the old and new treatment paradigms—medications, cortisone injections, viscosupplement injections, nerve blocks, epidurals, perineural superficial injections, or RIT. But in the acute injury phase of healing, I try to avoid giving patients an anti-inflammatory medication in most circumstances.

After I have established a diagnosis and begun to shut off a patient's pain, I next work to help him manage his injury going forward to avoid further problems. This was the case with Bettina, who was a recreational golfer in her late forties. She had come to me because her right knee hurt, and she was beginning to experience pain in her lower back. I did a physical exam, looked at her x-rays, and examined her with diagnostic ultrasound. She had moderate arthritis in her right knee and was beginning to show signs of facet joint syndrome in the right quadrant of her lower back.

It is always difficult to tell someone he is developing a degenerative disease that is going to impact his life. I started by saying, "You're here with pain in your knee, and you have x-rays showing evidence of arthritis. Your knee pain is most likely from the arthritis, and your lower back pain is most likely the result of limping from the knee pain going untreated. If my current diagnosis is correct, here are the options to treat your pain." First, I treated her facet joint problem through osteopathic manipulation. Since she had inflammation, with some fluid in the knee joint that needed to be removed, I suggested draining the fluid, then giving her one steroid shot.

On the next visit, Bettina told me she was feeling better. I responded, "Okay, your pain is under control now. You have this knee arthritis, which is beginning to affect your back. What do we do about it? For the time being, we will see if the manipulation, with some physical therapy, helps control your lower back pain. One way we can manage your knee is with a drug that's covered by your insurance—it's called a viscosupplement. Your other option, for both your knee and your lower back, is prolotherapy. Which option is best for you?" Like a lot of my patients, Bettina chose the treatments covered by her insurance. I encouraged her to keep up those treatments as long as they proved effective. If either loses its effectiveness, then I will discuss prolotherapy and other forms of RIT with her.

DYNAMIC STABILIZATION FAILURE AND POSTURAL DECOMPENSATION

What if Bettina didn't keep up with the viscosupplement injections or the healing process was arrested by life circumstances or another illness? What if Bettina was unable to go through the normal progression of recovery, from rest to physical therapy to regular, moderate exercise? Then her arthritic knee pain might not only become chronic, but also start to affect and inhibit larger and larger areas of her kinetic chain, as happened with Gretchen.

If a patient with pain and reflex inhibition is not treated properly, there is a chance they may go into dynamic stabilization failure.[11] Researchers have done experiments where they would take eight milliliters of fluid and inject it into a patient's knee. Now, that is a small amount compared to what I often take out of an arthritic joint. Within eight hours of injecting the fluid, weakness in the thigh muscle, which is responsible for holding the kneecap in the middle of the joint, is measurable. So if you have arthritis, and you develop a swollen knee because you went out and golfed or gardened too much, or you slipped and fell and banged your knee on the ice, the pain and swelling could be enough to start inhibiting muscles around that joint. This could lead to more dysfunction and a downward spiral. If this happened to Bettina, because the thigh muscle is no longer able to do its job, her problem might go from simple initial arthritic pain, to wear and tear on the back side of the kneecap where the cartilage is. Left untreated, that anterior knee pain could become patellar femoral pain syndrome, which causes the patient to start limping, then to have problems getting up and down steps. Long term, it could lead to additional arthritis behind the kneecap called chondromalacia. In the short term, it can lead to back pain, hip pain, and ankle pain.

The static stabilizers of the joint—comprised of the joint structure itself and the capsular ligaments that connect one end of the joint to the other—don't move voluntarily. Their job is to connect our bones together. The dynamic stabilizer is a muscle that both stabilizes and moves the joint, and also helps other muscles contract. If the static stabilizer is compromised due to a ligament sprain, arthritis or another injury, the joint may not be as steady as it could be. Then, the dynamic stabilizers are forced to become the primary stabilizer. They can't do so indefinitely, and eventually start to fail. Then more distant, indirect stabilizers try to stabilize the area, and fail. This goes up and down the kinetic chain. David Reid, M.D., first wrote about this in the early 1990s.[12] The entire joint structure becomes too tight, and restricts the patient's ability to move. If this happens, I offer my patient the spectrum of effective treatments available to him at this point, particularly RIT treatments, and let him decide how he wants to proceed.

If someone, particularly an athlete, continues to train after being injured, and is already experiencing some degree of dynamic stabilization failure, he might also develop postural decompensation. In this instance other muscles, which have been compensating for the failed dynamic stabilizers, will cease to do so. Muscles can only compensate for so long and then they too will fail.

This phenomenon accounts for why one seventy-year-old patient of mine is a dedicated, active, healthy golfer with excellent posture, while another is hunched over and relying on a cane. If I can get the static stabilizers working again and reverse the reflex inhibition with regenerative healing, I can help many patients live longer, healthier more productive lives.

Like Gretchen, they will come to me saying, "It started right here, in my knee, but now my hip hurts, my ankle hurts, my thigh hurts, and I'm getting pain in the left side of my neck." It's all connected. In many cases, it's all related to the original injury or disease.

CHRONIC REGIONAL PAIN SYNDROME

Another problem that can come from any injury that doesn't heal properly is chronic regional pain syndrome (CRPS), type l, which used to be called reflex sympathetic dystrophy (RSD). It is another form of pathologic, chronic pain. It can happen from a bad ankle sprain, it can happen from a failed surgery. And yes, even if the surgery is done properly, the patient still can get it spontaneously. CRPS can sometimes be treated with RIT, and, later in the book, I will tell you about patients who experienced substantial relief from this malady.

AVOIDING LATER DISABILITY

The most common joint sprain in the body is the ankle joint. With that said, the stage may be set for disability early in life with a sprain as common as this. The conventional standard of care for a sprained ankle is to rule out a fracture, apply an ankle wrap, and tell the patient to take an NSAID. This standard of care is a perfect setup for creating a future disability because of chronic joint instability.

If you put a patient on an anti-inflammatory, it may impede his normal healing. This is compounded if you don't give him any exercises to return the strength and range of motion of his injured ankle back to normal. The muscles around the injured

---

The most common joint sprain in the body is the ankle joint. With that said, the stage may be set for disability early in life with a sprain as common as this.

---

ankle weaken through reflex inhibition, and the ligaments don't heal completely due to the NSAIDs. This can lead to a chronically unstable ankle, which the patient may end up spraining many, many times over the next few years. Ankle sprains leave 10–40 percent of patients with chronic ankle instability.[13] Over time that instability can disturb the functioning of their kinetic chains, lead to dynamic stabilization failure, and ultimately predispose them to develop arthritis and postural decompensation. That's just one common problem that can lead to surgery or the possibility of a chronic disability. With timely and proper treatment, using RIT and completing a comprehensive rehabilitation program, ankle instability can be corrected, thus helping to prevent possible future injuries and eventual disabilities.

Another common injury, a rotator cuff tear, can also predispose a patient for early disability. The old treatment paradigm for these tears are rest, anti-inflammatory medication, physical therapy, a shot of cortisone or other medication, and, if the patient still is experiencing chronic pain and/or disability, surgery. While most surgical studies report high patient satisfaction following initial recovery from surgery, re-tear rates remain unacceptably high, in the 25–40 percent range. Also, I have heard from a lot of my rotator cuff patients that they were not terribly happy with either their long-term outcome or the long haul it took to recover from their surgery.

Using regenerative healing procedures could make a huge impact on people with injured or degenerated rotator cuffs. In some instances, it could significantly improve short- and long-term patient satisfaction and prevent recurring injuries and pain.

THE SPECTER OF ARTHRITIS

I think about how so many of us in the aging baby boomer population—whether or not we are athletes—are getting to the age where we can expect to develop arthritis. All the statistics predict it is the baby boomer generation that's going to break the Medicare bank.[14] Arthritis is going to play a huge part, as will the number of joint replacement surgeries arthritis will necessitate. In 2008 over half-a-million knee replacement surgeries were performed in the U.S., costing about $15,000 each.[15] That totals eight billion dollars spent on knee replacements alone in one year. Of the over 500,000 knees and over 250,000 hips replaced each year, 90 percent of these are surgically successful.[16] But, in up to one third of the cases, patients are not completely satisfied with their outcome.[17] These surgeries also leave patients with the likelihood that, in ten to twenty years, they'll have to endure revision surgery which is often much less effective.

Another looming problem stems from today's early specialization of the young athlete. When I was a kid, we didn't specialize until we were much older. We played outside, and each season brought a new sport. We didn't pick just one until we were well along in junior high school or even high school. If you have a young child who is a baseball pitcher from the age of five, it is unlikely he will get out of high school without an injury. Kids always ran the risk of being hurt playing sports, but with specialization, the injuries seem to be more serious and the consequences more profound. Over a quarter of a million youth baseball injuries are treated by medical professionals every year.[18] Unless these injuries are treated well and thoroughly, they can lead to a predisposition to get early onset arthritis or significant joint instabilities requiring high-risk surgeries on our youngest athletes.

Injuries can be serious and need to be dealt with quickly and properly, before they get worse or contribute to a second injury in another part of the body. I have almost had to go on disability myself, so I know the consequences of acute injuries, which become chronic. Through this book, you will become more aware of how injuries can affect you, and what you can do to help yourself heal as well as you possibly can without surgery. My goal in this book is to arm you with the knowledge I have gained, knowledge that will allow you to have the best possible care and, consequently, the best possible outcome for any injury you might sustain.

CHAPTER FOUR
WHAT HAPPENS WHEN YOU ARE INJURED

You have fallen, or exercised too vigorously. Perhaps you reached too high to return that ball. You may have been in an auto accident. You could have twisted your ankle on a stone you did not see while walking. There are so many ways to be injured. What now? Bethany, like 25,000 people each day in the U.S., sprained her ankle.[1] While this is one of the most common injuries, there are many original stories I have heard about what caused the twist. Bethany's was caused by a fairly common occurrence: She was going down her friend's front steps. When she reached the thick welcome mat at the bottom, it caught and turned her foot. She was lucky she only sprained her ankle. Oftentimes this scenario ends up with the person breaking one of the bones in her foot or ankle. I saw Bethany almost two months after the injury. Like many injured people she had been doing self-care. "I didn't think I needed to see a doctor for a twist or sprain," she told me. "I am taking ibuprofen (or naproxen or aspirin) because it hurts. I looked up ankle sprains online. I rested, used ice, an ACE bandage, and elevated it. I did all it said to, and it's not really getting back to the way it was. It hurts if I walk very far, and I can't play tennis. So, I asked some friends and found you." I am now dealing with a patient who has had minimal-to-no treatment for an undiagnosed acute injury, which, since it occurred over six weeks ago, has become chronic.

It was obvious from Bethany's history that she didn't know about the new healing paradigm and had seriously interrupted her body's natural healing cycle. I was able, with a good physical exam and diagnostic ultrasound, to find the ligaments she had torn in her ankle. Because of the length of time Bethany had been untreated, and the nature of her underlying injury, I went directly to RIT. After her prolotherapy treatments, and appropriate physical therapy, Bethany was able to resume her usual activities. Her ankle needs to be checked periodically to be sure the ligaments remain strong and stable.

Bethany was fortunate that she came—at least eventually—to a doctor who knew about both the old and the new injury treatment paradigms. Many doctors do not yet know what healing is possible with all the methods you will learn about in this book. If Bethany had gone to one of the other doctors in my community, he probably would have followed the old treatment paradigm exclusively, because the new-paradigm treatments are not yet the accepted standard of care. Why you may ask? Because some of these treatments are not covered by insurance, and many of them require the doctor spend a good amount of hands-on time with the patient. Unfortunately for patients, the current corporatized medical establishment rewards doctors for being quick in treatment, rather than being thorough.

"Old-paradigm" treatment is the type of care of acute and chronic injuries or degenerative diseases that I used to teach and practice. A physician who practices this paradigm can be a specialist in family medicine, emergency medicine, internal medicine, pediatrics, sports medicine, physiatry, or orthopedic surgery.

While these doctors have the old treatment paradigm in

common, there are substantial differences in how each deals with an injury. Emergency medicine, internal medicine, family medicine, and pediatric doctors have been trained to be generalists, to provide the first line of diagnosis and care for a wide variety of illnesses and injuries. Most of these primary care physicians have little interest in providing the full spectrum of diagnostic and treatment care available to the musculoskeletal specialist. Physiatrists, sports medicine physicians, and orthopedic surgeons are specifically trained in the care of the musculoskeletal system. Most physiatrists are trained and specialize in diseases of the spine; sports medicine physicians specialize in the complete health care of athletes; and orthopedic surgeons specialize in the operative treatment of injuries. Approximately 90 percent of all sports injuries are non-surgical.[2] If surgery is necessary, a well-trained physiatrist or sports medicine physician can expedite a referral to the right orthopedic surgeon in his community.

Sports medicine physicians are also trained in the non-musculoskeletal aspects of sports health. Common examples include concussions, exercise-induced asthma, overtraining and fatigue, return-to-play issues after being sick or injured, nutrition, training, and conditioning. To become a sports medicine physician, one must complete a residency in family medicine, emergency medicine, physiatry, or pediatrics, and then a fellowship of one to two additional years of training specifically focused on sports medicine—the comprehensive care of the athlete's orthopedic, medical, nutritional, and wellness needs. Sports medicine physicians are trained to care for non-athletes such as people who wish to begin an exercise program, or someone who has sustained an injury at work or at home, is experiencing musculoskeletal pain, or is looking to improve his overall health.

The sports medicine physician's training is spent primarily in the office, in the training room, on the field, at mass participation events, and in human performance labs. Conversely, the orthopedic surgeon's sports medicine training is primarily spent in the operating room, emergency room, and hospital. An orthopedic surgeon may do a surgical sports medicine fellowship focused on gaining additional surgical skills in shoulder and knee arthroscopic surgery.

I still use many aspects of this paradigm in the conservative care with which I frequently begin treating a patient. Some parts are good, miraculous when you consider people who would be in wheelchairs without them. But compared to the new paradigm I have learned, exclusive use of this kind of treatment is limiting. Too many of my patients were not finding relief.

CONTINUING STORY OF AN ANKLE INJURY

If Bethany had gone to her primary doctor and said, "I'm a runner, and this ankle hurts. What can I do?" the canned answer is, "If it hurts, then don't do it." In other words, if it hurts, stop running. The worst thing you can ever say to runners is "stop running," because running is an important part of their identity, their leisure time pleasure, and their health. In sports medicine, it's the last thing we tell a runner. We may recommend that runners stop running temporarily, but we tell them they can cross-train or run in the deep-end of a pool instead to keep their cardiovascular and psychological conditioning in good shape while their ankle or other injury heals.

Early on in my career, during the nearly twenty years when I worked in the emergency room, I practiced the old treatment paradigm. The most common injury I would see would be someone hobbling in with an ankle swollen to twice its normal size. If Bethany had gone to an emergency room, the first step in the old paradigm would be to send her for an x-ray to determine whether the ankle had a break or fracture. Then I'd have one of the medical assistants elevate her leg, put an ice pack on it, and wait

---

The worst thing you can ever say to runners is "stop running," because running is an important part of their identity, their leisure time pleasure, and their health.

---

for the radiology results. If nothing was broken, I would have prescribed something close to the formula that Bethany found in her Internet search of rest, ice, compression, and elevation (RICE). Because I am a sports medicine specialist, I would have changed RICE to PRICES, adding "protection from further injury" and "safe return to normal activity" to the formula.

I would have wrapped her ankle in a compression bandage and sent Bethany on her way, advising her to see her family physician as soon as possible. At that time of my practice, had it been a particularly bad sprain, I might have suggested the use of non-steroidal anti-inflammatory drugs (NSAIDs) for the pain, and fitted her with a brace and/or crutches to help her get around.

A primary care doctor probably would do the same. He might suggest Bethany come back in a few weeks to be sure the ankle is healing properly. If she asked, or if the doctor had sports medicine training as part of his or her residency program, he might write a prescription for physical therapy to help strengthen the ankle after it is healed. If, upon later examination, the doc did not like the way the ankle was healing, he might send her to a sports medicine doctor or to an orthopedic surgeon.

HAMPERING HEALING

The first thing Bethany did when she got injured was to reach for a NSAID. This immediately interferes with her body's initial healing process. NSAIDs are prostaglandin inhibitors. All different types of prostaglandin are produced from fatty acids and influence a variety of bodily functions, including inflammation, pain signals, and the maintenance of tissues. When you sprain your ankle and it becomes very painful, swollen, red, and warm to the touch, that's due to the early release of prostaglandin. If you inhibit prostaglandin in the early healing phase of an injury, you are limiting the scope and impact of that healing stage, and thereby all the latter healing stages. You are hampering the remodeling that can occur in that tissue. If you inhibit prostaglandin in the early healing phase of an injury, you limit the "stage" for the remodeling that can occur in that ligament. The larger the healing stage, the greater the potential for a completely healed ligament. If you put NSAIDs into the mix, you literally block your body's ability to produce the best outcome. A study called the Kapooka Ankle Sprain Study,[3] conducted by the Australian army in the late 1970s, is referenced in many medical journals. In this study, they took recruits who had ankle sprains and put half of them on an NSAID and half on a placebo, and got them back to marching as soon as each recruit was able. The study was promoted as proof that NSAIDs work because the recruits on medication were able to get back to marching sooner with less pain and less swelling than the patients on the placebo. But surprisingly, at the end of the study, long before doctors understood the negative ramifications of anti-inflammatories on healing, the group that received the placebo demonstrated fewer long-term problems. The doctors found in their post-study examination that the recruits who received the placebo had much more stable ankles. Study subjects taking the NSAID had a 25 percent rate of recurrence of sprained ankles.[4] Consequently, that same ankle sprain study is now being used as evidence to show that NSAIDs are actually harmful to the healing of a ligament.

Once I explain why we don't want patients to use NSAIDs during treatment, some become zealous about not using them. Bob, a young basketball player, fell into this category. He observed, "I used to take NSAIDs after I sprained my ankle, and it took about four days for the pain to get better. Now I don't take the NSAIDs, and it still takes four days to get better! That medication really just covered up my symptoms." I tell patients who are on chronic NSAIDs—for instance, an arthritic patient who comes to see me for some form of RIT—that if the only thing RIT can do is get them off their NSAIDs, it's potentially life saving. Twenty-five thousand people a year die from gastrointestinal bleeds and related complications from chronic NSAID use, and that number does not even take into account all the heart problems these drugs can precipitate.[5] According to a recent Danish study of over one million patients, patients taking ibuprofen, diclofenac, and Cox-2 inhibitors had a significantly greater risk of cardiovascular deaths, strokes, and heart attacks compared to those not taking any NSAIDs.[6] The possible exception was naproxen sodium, which was relatively neutral when it came to cardiovascular risk compared to those not taking NSAIDs. The Cleveland Clinic is conducting a long-term study of their population to ascertain whether the Danish study actually reflects cause and effect.

Back when I was doing orthopedic fracture care, I noted that most of the well-trained orthopedic surgeons were not using NSAIDs for fractures. They were using acetaminophen with codeine or some other narcotic to deal with a patient's pain. The major problem in using NSAIDs was the incidence of nonunions where the fractures didn't heal all the way. In that instance, the patient ended up having to go back to the orthopedic surgeon many times and often ended up needing some kind of surgery to fuse the bone together.

But while these progressive physicians had stopped using anti-inflammatory drugs for fractures, they still prescribed NSAIDs for tendinitis and sprains. There is now sufficient research showing that NSAIDs have the same adverse effect on healing other tissue types that contain collagen as they do on fractures.[7] They also appear to slow the tissue healing process. If there are signs of excessive inflammation and pain in a patient who has a bad sprain or a bad tendon injury, it is sometimes necessary to use NSAIDs, but the initial inflammatory healing stage should pass first. This means waiting five to seven days after the onset of the injury to use them.

OTHER MEDICATIONS WHICH COULD HARM HEALING

There are other commonly used medications suspected of interfering with healing, or even of exacerbating joint, tendon, and ligament problems. I recently wrote a letter for Brad, a patient whose doctor had given him very high doses of statins almost a decade earlier because Brad had a family history of high cholesterol, although no one in his family had died of heart disease. Normally, you put a patient on a statin dose of 20 milligrams and his LDL (bad cholesterol) will go down nicely. If he is resistant to statins, his doctor might raise the dose to 40 milligrams. Well, Brad had been up to 80 milligrams per dose. He had experienced severe fatigue and cognition problems. He had developed what's called "brain fog," which interfered with his ability to concentrate or recall. He had poor short-term memory. Previously a very quick thinker and talker, he had felt like everything was slowing down. He had aches and pains all over his body, his joints were hurting, and his tendons were falling apart. Having a medical background, he had taken himself off the high-dose statins. Within a few weeks, Brad's mental clarity had returned, but his tendons were still shot.

When I first saw him, he basically had pain all over his body. I worked on a couple of areas with RIT, and it helped him, but I hadn't seen the normal response I would expect. Brad had seen probably a dozen neurologists over the years, and none of them would admit there's a connection between statins and nerve and tendon disease. Yet he found a number of articles supporting his experience on MedLine and the Cochrane Database, important medical resources written for physicians.[8, 9] These are the databases that physicians rely on for researching the medical literature.

Candice is a patient I treated for one of the worst cases of frozen shoulder I have ever seen. I'll tell you more about her later in the book. She told me she had been a healthy, athletic person until a year before when a doctor prescribed a fluoroquinalone class of antibiotic for a persistent sinus infection. A number of weeks after taking the drug she began having multiple problems, including the one with her shoulder. Candice attributes her problems to taking the antibiotic and is active online with thousands of other people reporting the same sort of experience.

Another patient in my practice, Lou, came to us because he was told that both of his hips needed to be replaced. He believed his problems began about a decade before he saw me, when he was snorkeling and was stung by a sea urchin. The doctors treating him gave him a fluoroquinalone, which he took for a month. The swelling in his hand did not go down, and he had to have hand surgery. Shortly after, he began to have pain in his Achilles tendon. Five years later, he contracted methicillin-resistant *staphylococcus aureus* (MRSA), and was given another strong, intravenous (IV) antibiotic. He recovered from the MRSA, but soon after began having problems with pain in his legs, arms, shins, and quadriceps muscle. He tried a variety of cutting-edge allopathic cures, as well as massage, acupuncture, chiropractic care, acupressure, physical therapy, and a variety of supplements.

Before his snorkeling accident, Lou had been a very active person who had been training, in some fashion, six days a week since he was eighteen years old. He told me that he took great care of his body. When we examined his hips, we agreed that the right one will need to be replaced, but we hoped that we could save his left one through stem cell treatments. In the interim, we have been treating his other pains with PSI and other forms of regenerative injections. He has reported feeling relief from the treatments he has already had.

Lou told me, "There are a lot of people who depend on me, both in my family and in my businesses. I still look like I'm in good physical condition because I push myself to keep going. I am only fifty-seven years old. I want to be able to walk easily again, to ride my bike, and to do other simple things that I have always enjoyed. If my story can stop one person from having the same experience I have had, then I will feel I have done my job."

Lou also told me that what offended him greatly were the attitudes of most doctors he saw about his problem. They did not believe him. He recounted that his dentist "blew him off" when he first told him. Now, Lou said, that dentist won't prescribe fluoroquinalone because he saw what happened to Lou.

As Lou reports, most doctors do not believe there is a connection between fluoroquinalone and tendon and ligament pain. I'm not so sure. I have a history of tendon problems, and every time I've been to Honduras—seven times—I ended up having to take this type of antibiotic for "Montezuma's Revenge." I wonder if that has anything to do with my chronic tendon problems. Maybe this is a universal effect, or perhaps this is a genetic issue that only affects certain patients exposed to the drug.

Systemic steroid drugs can also contribute to one disease that has a profoundly negative effect on the bones.[10] This disorder, known as fatty liver changes, can actually cause the hip bone to die. I will tell you a story about a patient I have treated for this disorder in Chapter Nine.

Many people with chronic pain are prescribed narcotic pain medication that enables them to live with the pain. Such drugs, taken over time, can cause dependence and in some, addiction, and all the side effects that come with this. There are times when any one of these medications may be necessary and helpful. But, taken too long or by someone whose system cannot handle them, they can have a negative effect that might eventually outweigh the positive. There are risks and benefits with all medical procedures. The educated consumer needs to weigh them carefully.

MEDICATIONS THAT MAY HELP

Doctors practicing the old paradigm put their emphasis on treating musculoskeletal problems with medication. Why? Many patients would prefer to take a "magic pill," hoping to affect a cure with as little effort on their part as possible.

There are many medications to help with pain, inflammation, arthritis, and other disorders. Like the medications discussed in the previous section, they all have good points and bad. A patient comes to me with severe pain, swelling, and obvious signs

---

Many patients would prefer to take a "magic pill," hoping to affect a cure with as little effort on their part as possible.

---

of inflammation in an arthritic joint. I would drain the fluid out, and then consider putting a steroid shot in. How many times would I do that? Usually not more than once, because there is evidence that the more steroids I use in a patient, the more I may be blunting his ability to react to the arthritic progression of pain. If someone is over fifty, or has been hard on his joints, or had earlier injuries, chances are good some arthritis is present. If I'm covering up his pain, and he is able to use his joint, it may degenerate more quickly. Through the miracle of cortisone, he can continue to go out and train for a marathon or work as a carpenter, going up and down the ladder forty times a day carrying a heavy tool belt. The pain steroid shots have alleviated may not come back until the arthritis is rekindled because the patient overdid it again, or the inflammation in the joint reared its ugly head six weeks, to six months, to a year later.

When someone presents with his first episode of arthritic joint pain, it's commonly a mild episode. Arthritis is episodic—it may not come back again for a long time. Once the joint starts to degenerate at a more moderate pace, the inflammatory process may reappear much more often. Eventually, as the arthritic knee becomes end stage, you can do steroid shots in those joints all day long; it's not going to help pain that is coming from the joint being bone on bone. Then the patient is off to stem cell treatment or surgery. If I am talking about an active population, I think it's an accurate statement to say that giving a patient more than one cortisone injection each year in a weight-bearing joint puts the joint at risk for advancing arthritis quicker than if I treat it in other ways.

Viscosupplement injections have been a huge boon for patients previously receiving frequent intra-articular steroid injections, because they decrease the need for more frequent steroid shots. There are both synthetic viscosupplements and ones made from the comb of roosters. With this medication, I am able to get some patients off their anti-inflammatory medication altogether and only have to give them the viscosupplement shot once every six months. These are definite advantages, as is the fact that viscosupplement injections into the knee joint space and, in some states, the hip, are covered by insurance. The disadvantage of viscosupplement injections is that most physicians only inject into the knee joint space because of insurance reimbursement policies. I have been told a viscosupplement could be

injected more frequently into joint spaces, or into damaged ligaments or tendons, in the same way a prolotherapy solution can.
However, it would be much more expensive to use than simple
dextrose, which is the active ingredient in prolotherapy.

When this drug first came out, it was presented as a lubricant
for the joint to replace the pathologic joint fluid. Through reading and attending lectures, I learned the body rids itself of the
viscosupplement in a week, so I wondered how it could provide
six months' relief. My RIT colleagues and I theorized, and studies now support our theory, that there has to be an aftereffect. It
is most likely that in the process of the body's immune system
removing the viscosupplement molecule, the patient produces
many different growth factors, which precipitate a healing response in much the same way RIT does.

I said some of this in an orthopedic meeting where there
were only a handful of sports medicine docs trained like me. The
rest of those in the room were surgeons, most of whom viewed
RIT with skepticism at that time. I felt like I was a heretic, as I
imagine Louis Pasteur felt when he proclaimed that infections
are caused by microorganisms.

In my practice, I do use the old-paradigm treatments of
nerve blocks and epidural steroid injections to help with acute
and chronic nerve-related pain. Nerve blocks, which are injections of lidocaine, can be done anywhere a nerve is. In the old
paradigm, most nerve blocks are done on deeper nerves. I also
employ hydrodissection, also known as percutaneous neuroplasty, in which fluid is injected using high-resolution diagnostic
ultrasound to dissect the nerve away from the tissue compressing and entrapping it.

Like a good number of sports medicine doctors and physiatrists, I also use percutaneous needle tenotomy (PNT) to encourage healing of injured and degenerated tendons. I was taught this procedure in the early 1990s. In PNT, the physician makes at least twenty-five needle passes in a tendon to break up all of the diseased fibers and encourage blood flow. Used alone, I only observed about a 50 percent success rate with this procedure. After I began using RIT and combined it with PNT, I began to get substantially better results.

I also do epidurals, which are nerve blocks given in the epidural space in the spine, usually to help with arthritis or a disc problem. In an epidural, the injected medication affects inflammation or scar tissue and anything compressing or irritating nerves going from the spinal cord out to the periphery of the body. In the new paradigm, instead of high dose steroids, we are beginning to use other medications experimentally that will provide the same or even better outcomes for our patients who need the compressed or damaged nerve treated without the side effects of the steroids. Currently we are experimenting with PRP and low-dose (hypoosmolar) dextrose and ultra-low doses of dexamethasone, which seem to be working as well or even better than a traditional epidural steroid injection. I will use whichever old- or new-paradigm treatment my patient needs to help him heal in the best possible way with the least possible risk and fewest side effects.

SURGERY

In the old treatment paradigm, if all of the foregoing procedures do not give the patient sufficient relief, then it is time to see an orthopedic surgeon to consider surgery. Surgical treatment has performed miracles for millions of patients who, had they lived in the middle of the twentieth century or earlier, would have spent their lives bedridden or wheelchair bound. I have great respect for the outcomes so many people have had with surgery. Yet, I now know there are other options that can sometimes achieve the same or even better results with less downtime and fewer side effects and complications.

Trevor was a patient who came to me for another opinion about treating his meniscal tear. He asked, "What are all of my options, doc?"

I told him, "You do have a meniscal tear in your knee, and you also have moderate arthritis." Then I explained the RIT treatments I could offer him. He thought for a while, and then said, "I already saw two surgeons. They both want me in arthroscopic surgery tomorrow, and they say they can heal me. Why don't I just do that instead of doing all this RIT?"

I replied, "Well, you can do that. These are all treatment options; you just need to understand the risks and complications of each. Can you go through that surgery and do well, then return to work and to working out in a few weeks or a couple of months?"

Certainly, it's possible. This is a common outcome for young guys in the NFL who have a meniscal tear; the surgeon goes in and trims that little piece out, and the player is literally back on the field in a week. He does great because he didn't have any arthritis, he was in top physical condition, and the surgeon just removed a small flap of cartilage that was getting caught in the knee when he moved. The doctor didn't need to go into the area of the meniscus that's really responsible for all of the cushioning. In this sort of case, surgery seems like a miracle procedure. But if my patient already has some arthritis in his joint, the mere act of putting a surgical instrument in there can aggravate the arthritis. The increased inflammation can be severe and unre-lenting and it can take a very, very long time to calm down. It's kind of like taking your hand and putting it in a hornet's nest and stirring up the nest. Even though the surgery is done perfectly, you could be miserable for many months to a year or so waiting for the inflammation to calm down.

After surgery, if a patient has this complication, his doctor will likely give him a steroid shot or viscosupplement injection. May-be he'll come to me, and I'll do prolotherapy, PRP, or PSI to calm down the joint. Eventually, as time goes by, the pain may finally calm down. While there are no hard statistics available, orthope-dic surgeons typically tell patients anecdotally that arthroscopic surgery is only successful about 50 percent of the time for a me-niscal tear. As I'm going down a patient's history, and I see they had arthroscopic surgery for something in their knee, I'll ask, "How did that go?" It seems that way fewer than 50 percent of patients with a history of arthritis say it went swimmingly well.

I told Trevor that I know many progressive surgeons who commonly try to talk an arthritic patient out of doing the surgery. They'll suggest viscosupplement injections, and physical thera-py, and surgery only if nothing else has succeeded. Research is proving the validity of this view. In 2013, there was an article in the *American Journal of Sports Medicine* which demonstrated that, if a little more than 45 percent of the posterior meniscus is removed, it will lead to significant joint instability, possibly put-ting a much greater load on the joint surface and thus accelerat-ing arthritis.[11] More frequently, I am seeing patients who tell me surgeons are suggesting joint replacement for cartilage tears, even with patients as young as their forties. I ask those patients why, and they tell me, "I have arthritis, and he doesn't want to do a scope. He said it's not going to work."

It would appear these old-paradigm practitioners are going right from saying they are not getting the results they want from doing an arthroscopic surgery to saying that joint replacement is the way to go. They know that up to 90 percent of their patients do pretty well with joint replacement, at least in terms of surgical success. I told Trevor that I understand the surgeons' thinking. Most surgeons don't know about prolotherapy or don't believe PRP is effective because the literature has not yet shown it's helpful in healing meniscal tears. I and other new-paradigm doctors are commonly healing such tears. There's just not yet a pile of articles to show that it really works.

JOINT REPLACEMENT

When absolutely necessary, I do send patients for joint replacement surgery. Like successful regenerative injection treatments, it can be life changing. The first joint replacement was performed in 1962. Prior to that time, people with advanced arthritis got around however they could—with the help of canes, crutches, wheelchairs. However, like the medications I discussed earlier, replacement surgery has its good and bad points. As I have previously noted, 90 percent of joint replacements are considered surgical successes, but about one-third of patients are dissatisfied with their joint replacement. The current generation of joint replacements lasts ten to twenty years, depending on the size of the patient, how well he takes care of himself, and his general health. Then the joints have to be replaced again, and that can be a more difficult surgery with an even worse satisfaction score. My patients also ask me about the newest prosthesis available. I remind them that we won't know if new joint replacement models and procedures are better than what now exists until there is a proven track record, perhaps twenty years from now.

There have been a lot of new developments with joint replacement technology. While initially they were only available for the knee and hip, they are now also made for the shoulder, ankle, wrist, fingers, and toes. But all of these new treatment methods may not be as benign as a doctor or the advertising makes them out to be. For instance, consider hip resurfacing, which looked like it was going to be a great technique to offer a younger patient who needed a hip replacement, allowing him to keep his leg bones, which are capped with metal that fits into an artificial metal hip socket in the pelvis.

What happened—and evidently the manufacturers knew this was a risk—was the metal would grind and start to shave off little pieces, which leeched metal into the patient's bloodstream.[12] The metal used was cobalt, a substance that can precipitate heavy metal poisoning. This happened to thousands of patients who had this surgery.

I've heard nightmare stories from joint replacement patients who took six months to two or three years to heal, sometimes needing additional surgery, other times ending up in chronic pain at the end of the healing process. It's one of the risks of any surgery. Everything can be done perfectly, and you can still end up with chronic pain. I see it every week in my practice. When a patient is in chronic pain, the surgeon is out of his usual options. He may suggest revision surgery if he thinks that might help. Otherwise, he will send the patient to a pain management program that will help him learn to live with the pain, or give him lifelong medication to suppress the pain as much as possible.

CHAPTER FIVE
MANAGEMENT OF INJURIES

New-treatment paradigm practitioners treat patients in ways that will not only help them regain their health and physical function, but also help them keep it. The practice of functional management of injuries was developed in the 1990s, and allows the patient to maintain as much mobility as possible while he heals, rather than trying to heal through immobilization. To this end, new-paradigm practitioners take advantage of a wider range of treatments than their old treatment counterparts. Some of these techniques are so new they are evolving on almost a monthly basis. Others have existed for more than a hundred years, but because of time and financial considerations, have been largely abandoned by most physicians. Functional management utilizes these old-paradigm treatments, and also takes into consideration how the kinetic chain affects the progression of injuries. Thus, it can help protect against reflex inhibition, dynamic stabilization failure, or postural decompensation. The new treatment paradigm allows injuries to heal more naturally, with motion and along the lines of stress. This can reduce formation of scar tissue, which in itself can cause subsequent problems by irritating nerves, limiting normal motion, and causing pain.

OSTEOPATHIC MEDICINE

Generally, osteopathic medical schools emphasize a more integrative approach to medicine, as well as train their students in assessing the physical structure of the body. They teach manipulative skills that can bring the body into better alignment. Aside from this extra training, doctors of osteopathy (D.O.) and doctors of medicine (M.D.) get the same education in anatomy, physiology, microbiology, and pharmacology. Today, D.O.s specialize in all forms of medicine, and many rarely utilize the manipulative skills they have learned.

As a sports medicine specialist, I have had ample opportunity to use my manipulation skills, and developed some reputation at the residency program where I used to work. I would walk into an examining room accompanied by an entourage of medical students and residents who had not been taught these techniques. One patient, some years later, recalled jokingly, "You walked in with your white coat on and all these students behind you, and I told you my story and you laid your hand on me, and when you were finished I felt cured. Then you left the room as quickly as you came."

While my osteopathic training did not really make me into the "miracle worker" that patient teased me about, it did teach me that form serves function, and that the symmetry of the human frame is specifically designed to keep the eyes level. The human body will adapt in order to accomplish this. Humans have a great ability to compensate our postural needs to the environment, whether we're standing on an uneven surface or walking across rocks on a mountain range. But with some people that ability to adapt is not present from birth; with others it is lost through chronic injury and postural imbalance. We become asymmetric, which causes joint dysfunctions.

By adulthood, almost everyone has minor imperfections that cause the body's symmetry to be lost and dysfunctions to occur. Some come from the aforementioned; others from the way an adult's body has developed, such as a person with really weak ankles, or underdeveloped legs, overly large breasts, or a long, thin neck. Once the body's ability to compensate for these dysfunctions is lost, the patient starts to get symptoms. For example, if you have a short leg on one side, your pelvis will rotate forward to try to level out the other side. When that hip rotates,

---

> By adulthood, almost everyone has minor imperfections that cause the body's symmetry to be lost and dysfunctions to occur.

---

it causes tension changes in the back muscles and the stomach muscles, and a little rotation that transmits to the spine and sacroiliac joint. Left untreated, these can all lead to problems later.

Osteopaths use many different forms of manipulation to attempt to return the person to symmetry. The kind most people know about is the spine being cracked like some chiropractors do. Obviously, this is a direct form of manipulation. In forms of indirect manipulation, the doctor's hand is not even touching the patient, or is very, very lightly touching the patient, and thus trying to influence the joint motion. Sometimes manipulations work. Other times the patient is not capable of holding them or cannot be adjusted due to severe muscle imbalances.

Bernadette was one such patient. She had sustained a concussion with a neck injury playing rugby. While her concussion resolved naturally, she still had a lot of neck pain. She tried a variety of manipulative techniques including cranial sacral therapy. This is a popular form of therapy that stems from osteopathic teachings, and is designed to normalize the flow of cerebral spinal fluid between the cranium and sacrum, as well as to aid in direct and indirect manipulation of joints between the cranium and sacrum. Although I tried a series of manipulations with her, they did not work. Fortunately, regenerative injection treatments gave her the relief she sought.

Many of the patients who seek relief from pain have tendons or ligaments that are too tight. Tension is frequently the cause, as it was with Cynthia. A graphic artist, she would spend hours with her body in an asymmetric position while drawing. Over time, the tension of her positioning made her muscles tighten, then her ligaments and tendons. This pulled some of her neck vertebra out of alignment. She developed neck pain that would often trigger a headache. She came to me when her symptoms were quite new and, because of her timing, I was able to re-align her neck. I also prescribed physical therapy, and the therapist, through myofascial work (which I will describe later in the chapter), was able to ease the tension in her shoulders and neck. Cynthia experienced relief from her symptoms. If she continues to exercise the area and watch her position when she draws, I am hopeful she will not need further treatment.

More difficult to treat are patients who are too loose. I worked recently with Scott, who had a history of genetically loose ligaments. He had been water skiing and he fell. The rope jerked his arm and stretched out his shoulder capsule even more than it already was. It tore the cartilage in his shoulder joint called the labrum. He was looking at surgery, but because of his pathologic looseness, the surgery had a poor prognosis. Scott could have ended up losing function and being in chronic pain for the rest of his life.

I did three PRP treatments for him, and he was back to normal. He felt like his injured shoulder was now tighter than the other one, and he was looking forward to doing more waterskiing. Before he could return to the sport he loved, he was helping set up the stage at a high school play, lifting pretty heavy boxes, and working really hard. At the end of this project, Scott's shoulder was a bit sore and he felt like it had loosened up some again. Sure enough, it had. Patients who have genetically loose ligaments will always loosen back up again if they do too much. Then it is back to PRP or off to surgery. They need to be careful of how they exercise and what they do physically if they want to maintain a pain-free body.

Osteopathic manipulation can be used to restore normal posture, spine position, or joint position, and thereby, function. If successfully treated, a patient would be in good, neutral alignment and have balance between the muscles in the front and back of the body. He would be able to maintain his compensation mechanisms to keep his eyes level in most situations.

Once a patient is realigned, osteopaths are trained to try to influence the body's ability to maintain that symmetry using postural analysis, biomechanical assessment and/or gait analysis to determine appropriate methods to help the patient. I will discuss these shortly.

The first osteopathic medical school was formed after the Civil War, by a disgruntled M.D., Andrew Taylor Still.[1] During that war, you were judged to be a good doctor by how quickly you could saw off a man's limb to prevent gangrene. After observing this mode of medicine, Dr. Still searched for other ways to help patients. While he knew he could not cure infection with manipulation, he found there were many maladies that could be helped by these techniques. The methods he used developed into osteopathic medicine. The osteopathic medicine model is a combination of identifying physical dysfunctions then correcting them through manipulation while also utilizing standard medical analysis and care, as well as surgery.

CHIROPRACTIC MANIPULATION

As I have become more involved with practicing regenerative injection treatments, and, consequently, had less time to use other methods, I often refer patients to other osteopaths or to chiropractors for manipulation. Chiropractic manipulation stems from osteopathic manipulation. The first chiropractor, Daniel David Palmer of Iowa,[2] was not enamored with all the medical training an osteopathic doctor had to do; he was only interested in learning and applying manipulation techniques. So he broke away from the osteopathic profession and started the first chiropractic training program. The early teachers at chiropractic schools were osteopaths. Many of the techniques that chiropractors use today are osteopathic techniques. There's a lot of crossover between osteopathy and chiropractic manipulation. I have great respect for good chiropractors who work as part of a clinical team to successfully treat a patient.

PHYSICAL THERAPY

Most old-paradigm doctors don't immediately think of physical therapy (PT) as necessary for injuries or helpful for chronic pain. Instead, they are inclined to dispense medication or refer the patient to an orthopedic surgeon. I am a solid advocate of good physical therapy, with an emphasis on "good."

When hospitals and insurance companies began to corporatize and micromanage the field of medicine, they looked at physical therapy as a business. In analyzing its component parts, they determined that most patients who go through a physical therapy department improved about 50 percent.[3] To achieve this 50 percent improvement, there needs to be very little in the way of hands-on, skilled care. After corporate bean counters realized they could make the same amount of money with this model and get some results, they adopted it. Consequently, the role of the physical therapist shifted into that of an evaluator who diagnoses the injury and lays out the therapy plan, which a minimally skilled physical therapy assistant (PTA) carries out. There is very little manual therapy offered or performed, and one PTA may supervise three to four patients at a time. This model saved hospitals and insurance companies a lot of money compared to the former system, which required each skilled therapist to spend thirty minutes with a patient doing direct care. There are still some physical therapists that are gems in corporate, hospital-based settings. However, if your goal is to heal 100 percent and return to pain-free function, in my opinion you will much more likely reach this goal in a top-notch, privately owned physical therapy facility where the owners know the difference between these two models.

The direct patient care model is still used by physical therapists trained in Canada and Australia, as well as with ones in some of the private facilities in this country. All of these good therapists are trained in some form of myofascial release technique, such as active release technique (ART), Graston technique, and others. They also use forms of dynamic stabilization training—such as functional movement screening (FMS)—balance, taping, and other techniques to both bring relief and healing. Myofascial release, such as ART, combines range-of-motion work with tissue contact. The concept is to shorten an injured muscle, tendon, or ligament through movement, until the therapist can distinctly feel the area of restriction. Then the therapist creates tension from that area up the kinetic chain. At the same time, the practitioner stretches the muscle under his thumb and lengthens the muscle out until he gets a release from the damaged tissue. When this happens, the therapist may feel "pops" and "cracks" under his thumb, and knows he has separated areas of connective tissue that had become stuck together, causing pain and stiffness.

Across the board, my patients are happier with these types of therapies. At one point, when I was running the sports medicine training program, I designed a research project where we sent all tennis elbow patients who had failed PT, cortisone shots, and bracing to ART treatment, and about 35 percent needed nothing more. This type of myofascial release work has become part of the treatment paradigm I now use, especially for soft tissue injuries.

Myofascial release grew out of trigger point therapy, which was written about by Dr. Janet Travell,[4] President John F. Kennedy's personal physician. Dr. Travell first used the term "trigger point"[5] to describe a painful point in muscle or fascia that did not correspond to a particular trauma, inflammation, degeneration, or infection. This point feels like a nodule, is painful, often causes the muscle to twitch when it is touched, and can be responsible for pain referred to other areas connected to the muscle that contains the trigger point. Most other forms of myofascial therapy were developed from Dr. Travell's theories. Until recently, practitioners did not agree what constituted a trigger point.

Jay Shah, M.D.[6], who works with the National Institute of Health (NIH), finally resolved this issue using both biochemical analysis and electron microscopy. According to Dr. Shah, a trig-

---

I think trigger point therapy, physical therapy, and other ancillary fields of musculoskeletal medicine are all useful for the new healing-paradigm practitioner.

---

ger point is an irritated muscle spindle that can be relaxed from its hyperactive state by inserting a needle into it. This injection or "needling" procedure was classically taught and performed with lidocaine. The physician must target the primary trigger point and relax it. This will resolve the secondary trigger points as well.

Dr. Travell said she believed the trigger point indicated problems further up or down the kinetic chain. Before her death, it is reputed that she told some of her closest associates she believed prolotherapy might be able to deal better with such underlying problems. She asked them to find the connection between trigger point work and prolotherapy.

I have noticed in perineural superficial injections (PSI) that when I put a shallow needle into an area where the nerve feels a little swollen, it's not uncommon for the needle to touch the muscle below it, and cause a big muscle trigger point twitch. Consequently, I see a correlation between PSI, trigger point therapy, and other superficial anesthetic injection techniques. As researchers continue to find connections between superficial techniques and prolotherapy, it is very possible that Dr. Travell's hypothesis might be proven true.

I think trigger point therapy, physical therapy, and other ancillary fields of musculoskeletal medicine are all useful for the new healing-paradigm practitioner. Here's an example. Alicia came for prolotherapy treatments to her spine. When she came in, I found she had a lot of spinal dysfunction, due to ligament instability. She was in chronic pain, which a combination of osteopathic manipulation and prolotherapy corrected. The prolotherapy tightened up her ligaments and helped hold the neutral alignment she enjoyed. She was now pain free, but still stiff, resulting in problems with her muscles.

At this point, she was ready to go back and finally finish her physical therapy, which she had not originally been able to do because of chronic pain and reflex inhibition. When she started PT, the therapist found some areas that prolotherapy had tightened up too much. She got in there with myofascial work and loosened those tight areas. They are now back to normal, and Alicia's stiffness and muscle pain are gone. Without this ancillary help, Alicia's healing would not have been complete.

While I feel almost everyone can benefit from physical therapy, the timing of it, and the type are of utmost importance. Remember that reflex inhibition only resolves when pain is gone. If someone suffering from this is forced into physical therapy too soon, this could increase pain and impede healing.

I see patients every week who have expended a lot of time and effort in physical therapy for a soft tissue injury. In my experience, now augmented by diagnostic ultrasound, I have found that if a good physical therapist has not significantly helped a patient in two to four weeks of work, the patient's soft tissue is torn, until proven otherwise. No amount, even of excellent physical therapy, will help that tissue heal if it has turned into a chronic injury. This is where RIT can make a huge, early difference. Once the tissue heals and the patient's pain drops by 80–85 percent, it is then time to finish physical therapy and help the person return to full function.

It is always best to start with early physical therapy goals and see how the person responds. While stretching and range-of-motion exercises can usually be accomplished safely and fairly soon after injury, strengthening exercises should be approached cautiously. I had one patient, Lucille, who was sent to vigorous PT too soon after a surgery to repair her knee. Her reaction to PT was so bad it was definitely a contributing factor in what became chronic regional pain syndrome, type 1. When I saw her, in order to start her healing, I had to suggest she rest without exercise or physical therapy until her pain had been reduced by over 80 percent. This took a year of intensive RIT work before she could return to PT. Following, she was able to consciously, gently resume some of her normal activities. Another patient, Kim, had headaches and migraines stemming from a bike accident when she was a girl. She reported in our first appointment that she had seen a cranial sacral specialist, and had undergone massage and physical therapy. These all increased her headaches. It was only through PSI that she began to experience relief.

Kinesio taping is a muscle treatment that is being used to help treat injuries and allow athletes to return to function earlier. The difference between kinesio taping and athletic taping is the athletic tape forms a splint that restricts motion. Kinesio tape is applied over muscles, does not restrict motion or function, and can stay on for more than twenty-four hours at a time. Although *The Journal of Orthopedic and Sports Physical Therapy* recently said, "There is little quality evidence to support the use of kinesio tape over other types of elastic taping in the management or prevention of sports injuries,"[7] athletes swear by it. Clinicians all over the world are using kinesio tape, and anecdotal evidence supporting its efficacy abounds.

PROTECTING INJURIES

Another difference between the old treatment paradigm and the way I practice now is in how I deal with protecting an injury. When I first got into sports medicine, the standard procedure was to cast a bad sprain for two to three weeks. Because of the stiffness after casting, it took six weeks for most patients just to get back decent range of motion. As I learned more, whenever possible I would put patients in boots and braces rather than casts. These give support, but allow for range of motion work, and give a patient the ability to take the boot or brace off, thus promoting natural healing and less loss of motion. Today, casts tend to be the exception rather than the rule for soft tissue injury management. Even in the case of a sprained knee, I prefer to put a patient in a brace with a hinge, which gives the ability to maintain the range of motion. This helps avoid significant quadriceps atrophy.

Braces come in two types: treatment and functional. Treatment braces are clumsier, sturdier, and more restrictive; the functional brace is lighter, made of nylon or neoprene, and has more straps. Emergency rooms are full of treatment braces and splints for every injury. Functional braces are the realm of the sports medicine doctor. They allow the patient to perform their rehabilitation program or, if far enough along in their therapy, to actually participate in their sport.

If I was prescribing range of motion work with a lateral structure, like the ligaments on the outside of an ankle, I would allow the patient to flex and extend his ankle in a straight line, but not to bend laterally, which would stretch the damaged ligaments. As the new ligament tissue is being laid down, proper motion allows the collagen to form more normally along the lines of natural stress, preventing a painful and dysfunctional scar from forming.

Evan was a young man who had sprained his knee ligament, was put in an immobilizer and given a pair of crutches in the emergency room. When he came into my office four weeks later, he had extensive quadriceps atrophy and a stiff knee, although the ligament he sprained was well on its way to healing. The first thing I did was to take him out of the immobilizer and put him in a knee brace with a hinge so he could work on his range of motion while the ligament continued to heal. Most of the time knee injuries don't need to be strictly immobilized to heal properly. The ligament or tendon can heal while the patient continues to use it, albeit in a modified fashion. Through range-of-motion work and quadriceps muscle strengthening, Evan was able to get his quadriceps and knee range of motion back in shape while his knee ligament continued to heal. This allowed him to avoid spending a good deal of time rehabilitating from quadriceps atrophy and severe joint stiffness caused not by his injury, but by his treatment.

GAIT TESTING AND LEG LENGTH

When evaluating a patient, like all good osteopaths and chiropractors, I carefully consider how he or she is built, and how the injury has affected his symmetry. A misaligned biomechanical structure can cause or exacerbate an injury. Restoring alignment should be the first step when initiating treatment. Physical manipulation is only one of the ways in which this can be accomplished.

In the sports medicine fellowship program I used to run, I scheduled lectures on biomechanical assessment, including both postural analysis, and attention to how a person moves. We taught our fellows how to do gait assessment, observing patients walking and running on treadmills, and identifying what's normal and what's not normal. If someone comes in with a cartilage tear on the inside of his knee, and has a really flat foot on that side, that's going to put more stress where the tear is. In such a case, it makes sense to fit him for an orthotic (a shoe insert) that will put him in a neutral position and help take enough pressure off of that knee joint so it can heal with the treatments that follow. But in a typical orthopedic, internal medicine, pediatric, or family medicine residency, they don't get that type of that training, so gait testing would be a completely foreign concept to them. A good sports medicine program will teach this, but programs vary. There isn't a mandatory curriculum that each sports medicine program around the country has to follow, so the design of any sports medicine program is predicated on the fellowship director, and how he was trained.

ORTHOTICS AND HEEL LIFTS

Evaluations of leg length difference are regarded differently depending on the doctor's specialty. An orthopedic surgeon is concerned about leg length only after someone has broken his leg, or has had a joint replacement. If there is less than one-inch disparity, the surgeon believes that the body will compensate just fine.

The osteopath who is taking care of someone with a bad back and finds the sacral base tilted may discover a significant leg length difference of about six millimeters. A sports medicine doctor or a podiatrist who is dealing with a leg length problem in a runner may notice a significant difference of three millimeters. When you run, your foot is hitting the ground about fifteen hundred times per mile. This could be enough to throw off the ankle, knee, hip, or spine. So the range of what's significant in a leg length difference evaluation depends on the criteria of the clinician who performs it. If you think you have a leg length difference or a postural issue, you should be looking for a doctor who's good at both orthotics and spine evaluations so he can work on both issues together.

If I'm thinking about giving someone a heel lift to equalize his sacral base, I would look at his feet first and see if he needs prescription orthotics. Orthotics can level out the subtalar joint right below the ankle as well as accommodate leg-length problems. If the subtalar joint is out of whack, it has far-reaching effects not only in our foot and ankle, but up the kinetic chain to our knees, hips, and back. If I prescribe a heel lift or orthotic, I ask the patient to see me for a reexamination in two to three years, because often the body starts making its own permanent corrections over time.

For example, Aaron had a very high instep that was beginning to put stress on his plantar fascia. I fitted him with custom orthotics, and that got rid of the stress. When I saw him two years later, he reported his problem had disappeared with regular use of the orthotics. However, they were beginning to wear. When I measured Aaron for a new orthotic prescription, I found a marked difference in both his instep and the rest of his foot. It was almost as though the orthotic or something else had allowed the rest of his foot to relax and normalize.

Putting an insert into a shoe may seem ridiculously straightforward, but it's important that you see an experienced clinician for this. There have been so many patients I've seen over the course of my career who have been injured by poorly made or fitted orthotics or heel lifts. I have seen them put in backwards, upside down, or in the wrong shoe. Harry was one such patient. Surprisingly, he had been wearing his orthotics in the wrong shoe for several months. I looked at him and asked, "How could you wear these?" And he said, "Well, the doctor didn't say anything when I put them in."

I can only assume the doctor was very busy and had not taken the time to check what Harry had done. He was fortunate he came to me for another injury as soon as he did, and that he mentioned his new orthotics. I've seen stress fractures from orthotics, and severe nerve injuries that extend all the way up into the hip. Too often a patient is given an orthotic and told to break it in, give it a month, and then he doesn't see the doctor again. So the patient thinks, "This is the way it's supposed to be," even if he is in more pain than he was before. The bottom line is that an orthotic should not make the problem worse. If it is, you should stop wearing it. Take the thing out and bring it back in to the doctor for a reevaluation.

BARE FOOT RUNNING

Bare foot running and intrinsic foot muscle training are relatively new healing paradigms for long distance runners who are prone to injuries. Their popularity started with a book, *Born to Run,* by Christopher McDougall, who, in a quest to figure out why he was so injury prone during his long distance running career, studied runners from all over the world.[8] He heard about the Tarahumara, a tribe of Mexican Indians, all barefoot long distance runners who ran a little differently than the typical American runner who had had a pair of shoes on his feet from an early age. McDougall discovered that these barefoot runners ran softly, with a shorter stride, landing on the midfoot instead of heel to toe like most American runners naturally do. I have found that when the gait cycle is changed in this way, some types of injuries can be healed and others avoided. But, when a runner tries to make this gait change too quickly, or does this change incorrectly, this new training regimen can be a source of additional injuries. If the transition to midfoot strike with a minimalist shoe is followed gradually, as described in the book, it may be a significant improvement for many runners.

ELECTRICAL STIMULATION, ULTRASOUND, LASERS, AND INFRARED THERAPIES

In physical therapy, electrical stimulation and ultrasound are routinely used during periods of acute pain in the immediate aftermath of an accident or injury to give some relief. I sometimes suggest that a patient with intense or chronic pain purchase a transcutaneous electrical nerve stimulation (TENS) unit for home care. The low-level electrical charge from such units helps to stimulate nerves and lessen pain.

Christina had been in a serious automobile accident in which she sustained shoulder, neck, knee, and ankle injuries, and a concussion. When I first saw her after the accident, I was unsure how well she could recover and return to her previous level of activity. I first sent her to physical therapy to receive a combination of electrical stimulation, therapeutic ultrasound, heat and cold therapy, along with some very gentle stretching and range of motion instruction. By her next visit, she had improved enough that I could make a more aggressive treatment plan that eventually brought her back to her pre-injury condition.

Ultrasound therapy is done with a machine that uses sound waves to generate heat within a part of the body. This helps loosen up tissues, thus allowing them to respond better to manual techniques, which relax tight joints or muscles. Ultrasound used without generating heat can help increase blood flow so inflammation or swelling is reduced.

I think both cold (class 3) lasers and, particularly, hot (class 4) lasers, have promise of potential therapeutic benefit when used properly. The difference between the two is in the wavelengths and, obviously, in the heat generated. While scientists can't yet fully explain how lasers work in therapy, there are a variety of theories. One is that, when directed into the body, a laser is a heat source which causes movement of the molecules in our tissues, and might release growth factors. Because of this very deep heat, lasers can alter biochemical processes and change tissue on a microscopic level. When used regularly, or after a regenerative injection treatment, laser treatment may help the body heal more efficiently. However, class 3 lasers can be used immediately after RIT. Because of the stronger heating effect of class 4 lasers, they should not be used until a month after treatment.

Electric stimulation, therapeutic ultrasound, and infrared light therapy all have fairly poor clinical research behind them, but they have been in use for decades to help reduce swelling, treat pain and spasm, and activate muscles that have not been used properly in a long time. Each of these therapies has its limited role, and, when combined together, they seem to have added benefits. I would consider them worthwhile adjuncts to try in individual cases and gauge how much benefit the patient thinks he is getting.

ACUPUNCTURE

Acupuncture works through the body's electrical nervous system by interacting with the superficial nerves, all the way to the deeper nerves in our bodies. Acupuncture not only affects the somatic nerves in our body, meaning nerves we can control with voluntary action, but also connects to the areas we can't voluntarily control, the sympathetic and the parasympathetic systems of our body. The sympathetic nervous system is extremely important in pain management, and if it becomes hyper-irritated, that can really send a patient who has an acute pain condition into a chronic, downward spiral. In my experience, acupuncture can arrest the acute pain and, more importantly, improve the autonomic nervous system to prevent or improve chronic pain at a deeper level. Many of my patients who have used the services of acupuncturists felt these treatments were beneficial.

FINDING GOOD PRACTITIONERS

I treated a patient, Hillary, whose experience illustrates the critical importance of finding good practitioners. Hillary had, eight years before, gone to a therapist because she had pain in her lower back. This therapist thought she had piriformis syndrome, a disorder caused by compression or irritation of the sciatic nerve by the piriformis muscle. In trying to treat it, he took his elbow and drove it into the bottom of her buttock, crushing her sciatic nerve against her pelvic bone. Hillary had immediately felt a burning, shooting pain down to her toes. She shouted, but he told her it was important for her therapy. When he let go, the pain she had felt did not subside, and she lived with it from that time on.

After I examined her physically, radiologically, with diagnostic ultrasound, and with electromyography (EMG) testing, I determined that her pain was coming from nerve damage. I started her on a course of perineural superficial injections, as well as percutaneous neuroplasty hydrodissection, in two different nerve areas. This treatment has given her the first pain relief she's had since that incident, and she is over 70 percent improved at the time of writing.

How well any ancillary treatments work depends on the ability and training of the practitioner, so it is critical to find the best therapist you can. The top therapists are hands-on specialists who have learned a lot of different manual techniques, even if they choose to specialize in one. Every time a patient comes in, the therapist is working with him directly, overseeing his exercise program and being sure the patient is advancing through his therapy goals from one phase to the next, back to full pain free activity.

Patients ask me where to find such therapists. Word of mouth is often the best way, but, what suits one patient's therapeutic needs may not suit another's. Ask your doctor and ask friends in the community, especially athletes or parents of a serious child athletes who have been injured. An athlete who's been injured and is trying to get back to the field of play will do almost anything to shave a couple of weeks off his therapy. He knows where to find the practitioners who get people better quicker.

When you have found a potential therapist, don't be afraid to ask questions. Ask about his training. Ask if he does hands-on work. Check if the therapist has a wellness program available when physical therapy is finished. Look at the facility in person and be sure it has sufficient equipment and space. Be sure the therapist will be the one treating you, or at least overseeing most of your treatment. If, during treatment, you feel the therapist is actually injuring you, you have every right to tell him to stop, and to leave if he won't. There is a certain amount of pain concomitant with deep-tissue work. Some people have a more difficult time with this, yet almost everyone is aware if something really feels wrong. It is at that point that you need to voice your concern.

I suggest patients follow the same approach when seeking any kind of ancillary help from a chiropractor, massage therapist, acupuncturist, or another kind of practitioner. I also suggest people don't do too many different methods at the same time. If you do, it can be difficult to judge what is really helping you. Again, remember, it is good to go from the least invasive end of the healing spectrum to more aggressive or invasive. This applies to massage and physical therapy, as well as to physician care.

Most of the methods I have introduced in this chapter have good, long track records. They have helped a lot of people overcome injuries and pain. However, they take more time on both the part of the patient and the physician. They will not give you the instant relief of a pain pill or an NSAID. Nor will they give you the side effects. They will encourage rather than hamper your long-range healing and return to full function. Whether you want to seek out the doctors and therapists who know them, and whether you want to dedicate the necessary time to using them, is ultimately up to you.

CHAPTER SIX
WHAT THE NEW HEALING PARADIGM OFFERS YOU

What will the new healing paradigm give you that your regular doctor hasn't already offered? Most important are a major difference in philosophy and cutting-edge healing options. New treatment-paradigm practitioners trust in your body's ability to heal itself, either naturally or by their giving you a push in the right direction. Sometimes that push is a small one: manipulation, good myofascial therapy, abstaining from or taking the correct medications for your stage of healing. Sometimes it is a stronger one, like a course of regenerative injection treatments. Given this push, treatment from a physician versed in the new healing paradigm, and good ancillary care, many patients who might have become incapacitated can return safely to full, healthy activity.

Old-paradigm practitioners largely rely on medication, therapy, and surgery to adequately treat injuries and chronic conditions. This kind of treatment sometimes fails to see the big picture, and to respond to it quickly enough, resulting in patients ending up in chronic pain. With many of the conditions I am discussing, timing of accurate diagnosis and of treatment is critical. If I am taking care of someone with bone-on-bone arthritis, there are fewer options than there are for a person who has mild arthritis and is just beginning to become symptomatic.

With the regenerative healing paradigm, I can do a great deal for the latter patients and possibly prevent them from ever needing a joint replacement. This new treatment paradigm can also help some patients nearing end-stage arthritis, usually through stem cell treatments.

In the last chapters, we looked at the old treatment paradigm, what it does offer and what it could offer. In this chapter, we will examine the differences both in philosophy and initial treatment between the old and new paradigms. The new paradigm has been developed through the work of doctors looking for methods that

---

What used to keep me up at night when I was only practicing the old treatment paradigm were the patients who didn't get better. I kept questioning why.

---

complement both traditional sports medicine and orthopedics. These physicians are doing both the research and the treatment necessary to establish two new specialties: integrative orthopedic medicine and interventional orthopedics. These specialties consider the underlying causes of chronic conditions—reflex inhibition, postural decompensation, and dynamic stabilization failure, among others. They also give patients a wider choice of treatment options, like regenerative injection treatments, in addition to techniques known to old-paradigm practitioners, but not widely used by many of them.

What used to keep me up at night when I was only practicing the old treatment paradigm were the patients who didn't get better. I kept questioning why. Was it biochemical? Was it hormonal? Did they have a genetic tendency to poor healing? Had they taken NSAIDs too early? Was their treatment brace or cast left on too long? Any of these things could contribute to healing results that left both me and my patient disappointed.

The more I learned about the new healing paradigm, the more I became convinced that not only were we doctors not using the full arsenal of treatments at our disposal, but also we were not always looking at an injury with the most comprehensive view. I became certain that it is imperative for doctors to consider the connections between all of the possible pain generators and either rule them in or out to make an accurate diagnosis, and, consequently, the best treatment plan. This takes time, and a deep understanding of both injury progression and the healing process.

HOW CAN I HELP YOU?

Patients can be treated very differently by doctors practicing the new rather than the old treatment paradigm. This begins with the initial examination. My first question to a new patient always is, "How can I help you?" And I have allotted time for him or her to answer fully. I need to know the history of his or her chief complaint.

Let's say my patient has a shoulder problem, one of the more common injuries I see in my practice. He would usually start his history by telling me when and how he hurt himself. I would then have him describe his pain using a scale from 1 to 10 (where 10 is the worst pain imaginable and 1 is hardly anything) when he is at rest, doing normal activity, or with more physical activities, like participating in a sport or gardening. Does his shoulder hurt all day long, or only with certain activities (like working out or lifting something over his head)? What makes it worse? Does anything make it better? How long has he had this injury? Has it changed over time? What are the restrictions his body has forced him to obey? Does his injury prevent him from being able to reach over his head, or behind his back? Is he able to groom his hair or get dressed in his normal manner? Pain and restriction of certain motions are both classic signs of shoulder impingement and/or a frozen shoulder.

Then I would find out how my patient has cared for his shoulder thus far. What did he do for self-care? Has he seen other doctors? If so, what have they prescribed? Has this patient had osteopathic or chiropractic manipulation, physical therapy, a shot of cortisone, or another type of medication? When I am doing my initial history, I focus on one specific injury at a time. I've learned the benefit of keeping the patient focused and the interview pertinent to the area most injured. Up to this point, what I have done is what any good physician with sufficient time allotted would do, or at least should do.

Then I will veer off from the normal. As an interventional orthopedic medicine specialist, I will encourage my patient to give me a bigger picture. For example, with our hypothetical shoulder problem, I would consider whether there is a neck problem that could be radiating pain to the shoulder. Does an adjacent area hurt? Is there a recurrent history of the problem? Has there been a change in general health? Has the patient been on some kind of new medication? I'll screen a patient's medical history and look for signs and clues that might suggest the pain is coming from or made worse by another source.

Sometimes, what I find astounds me. I have worked with patients who have been given high doses of medications suspected of causing problems with tendons and ligaments. I have seen patients wearing their custom-made orthotics upside down. I have treated a patient who got a hip fracture from a poorly made orthotic. I have worked with many patients whose dynamic stabilization failure was diagnosed as everything from mental or emotional problems to stress to fibromyalgia.

I still hear today from my patients that many doctors spend a lot more time looking at the diagnostic tests, the x-ray, or the MRI, than actually examining patients. I am told, "The doctor hardly touched me, doc, or didn't touch me at all." I get comments about my exam such as, "That was the most thorough exam of my injury I've ever had a doctor do." Another patient expressed it to me this way, "You can imagine, after seeing some of the pre-eminent specialists in the area I was extremely skeptical about what you could do. But you were the first doctor who actually listened to me and asked questions for thirty or forty minutes before even doing an exam. You had a completely different approach." This comes from my following the new paradigm of treatment.

I ask my patient what he thinks his problem is. Many patients do have an idea about what is wrong. They come in saying, "Doc, I hurt my rotator cuff," or, "Doc, I think I tore my labrum." They come in armed with information from reading, talking with other people—a coach, teammate, or neighbor—or browsing the Internet. They do try to self-diagnose, and often they have pre-set ideas. I like it when my patient has already put time and thought into what could be wrong with him. It means he is aware and involved in his own healing.

Some physicians don't share my view that it's perfectly fine for a patient to have his own ideas about what is wrong, or to suggest he thinks his shoulder pain could be coming from someplace else, like his neck. If your doctor is only focusing on your shoulder and does not want to hear about your neck, you need to tell him, "Hey, I'm having this neck problem, too—could the shoulder pain be connected to my neck?" If the doc won't discuss it, you should seriously consider finding another physician. From my perspective, the more the patient is armed with knowledge, the more he can be a participant in his health care, and that is a very important concept: medical awareness. Without medical awareness, it's more likely that you'll unquestioningly trust your doctor, and that can be dangerous.

I not only listen to my patient. I look at how he stands, walks, and sits. This is the beginning of my biomechanical and physical examination. Then I check his range of motion accurately. I test his manual muscle strength and grade it. I do special tests for ligament stability and joint integrity. I palpate where the pain is most likely coming from, and check the joint above and the joint below. I order and consider all relevant radiological studies. I often supplement them with diagnostic ultrasound. This sort of analysis is different from old-paradigm doctors who rely much more on radiological tests to make their diagnosis and generate their treatment plan. If I am going to offer a patient physical therapy or injection work, I have to be sure to pinpoint the problem and address it correctly.

I also consider the patient's lifestyle before making a diagnosis. What is his profession? Does he have a family? What kind of social activities does he enjoy? What is his activity level? Is he involved in a sport? Does he work out? How much time does he spend sitting, standing, walking, or moving? How is his general health? What medications is he taking? Remember how different kinds of medications affect your muscles, tendons, and ligaments, as well as other parts of your body.

AGE MATTERS

I consider my patient's age. For instance, Jerry came to me thinking he had a rotator cuff problem, which is a common cause of frozen shoulder. Jerry was twenty-three-years old, so I knew, statistically, it was unlikely that was his problem. Because of his age, I would suspect the cause of his painful shoulder to be tendonitis, an inflammation of the tendon. Rotator cuff injuries aren't that common in the young. They can develop from overuse or falling on the shoulder, but Jerry had not told me about a fall or increased activity. In a young person, even a rotator cuff injury will most often be cured just by relative rest and a focused home exercise program for a few weeks. Some younger patients may need an anti-inflammatory drug or some myofascial release, or physical therapy, but generally a painful shoulder is not a big problem. Young people who have this injury usually heal well.

If a patient is between the ages of twenty-five and forty, it is likely that he has developed a decreased blood supply to the end of the tendon where the injury started. In the beginning of the injury, any inflammation that was causing pain burned itself out within a few weeks. Then the tendon began to degenerate, so the stage was set for tendinosis, a chronic, diseased tendon. A patient with this will need more than rest and time to heal. Some forms of RIT would definitely be helpful.

In patients over forty—particularly those who keep overusing their degenerating tendons—I start to see the tendon suffer micro-tears. These small tears can coalesce and turn into a big macro-tear, which I can see with the help of an MRI or diagnostic ultrasound. A patient with this condition would definitely benefit from regenerative healing techniques. When a patient reaches his fifties or sixties, suffering with untreated or ineffectively treated micro-tears, and undergoes a slip or fall, or is in his car when it is rear-ended, the rotator cuff may rip more severely. In the old paradigm, it would be time for surgery.

In the new paradigm, even if surgery seems probable for a patient, I may still offer him some other options first. I might say, "You have time. RIT may not necessarily change the final outcome. You may still need surgery, especially if there is evidence of bony impingement causing the rotator cuff tear, but I think it would be worthwhile to try some other methods first and see if you can possibly avoid an operation. RIT has worked well for some of my patients with similar conditions and it carries less risk than surgery."

Surgery does have risks. I have cared for many patients who still suffered pain and had ongoing problems after surgery was completed. In some of these instances, it turned out their underlying problem was coming from undiagnosed, minor (or not so minor) tears of the surrounding tendons, cartilage, or ligaments. These patients might have avoided surgery if they had been examined with diagnostic ultrasound in addition to other radiological studies. After using ultrasound to make a definitive diagnosis, I would then have undertaken the proper form of regenerative injection treatment to most likely help them heal their conditions.

THE HEALING SPECTRUM

When I treat a patient, I believe in working through the healing spectrum, beginning at the least invasive end. When I first meet a patient, I rarely suggest RIT as the initial treatment. In general, I believe the less I have to do to help heal the problem, the better. My treatment strategy for patients whether they come in with an old injury, a chronic injury, a sub-acute injury, or a new injury, is to begin with a trial of the most conservative therapy they have not yet tried.

A good example is my patient Jeff, a student who rowed crew for St. Joseph's University in Philadelphia. He was eighteen years old when I first saw him. He had developed chronic low back pain. His mom saw a story on television about platelet-rich plasma (PRP) and brought him in to see me, requesting this therapy. I asked them what they had already tried. Who had he seen? Had he tried physical therapy? Did he have an MRI? Did he have steroid shots or an epidural? He replied that he had not tried any of these options.

I told him and his mother that we were going to take his treatment plan in steps, not rushing into anything that might not be necessary. I also explained I almost always try a course of prolotherapy before using PRP in the spine. I obtained his history, and did a thorough physical examination, determined his clinical diagnosis, sent him for x-rays and an MRI, and then got him going with physical therapy. He had some inflexibility in his back and hamstrings. I prescribed myofascial work at the same time as physical therapy. When I saw his MRI, it revealed a large herniated disc in his back. Still, the physical and myofascial release therapy worked after six weeks, and he felt about 85 percent better.

I determined he didn't need prolotherapy at this point. I wanted to let his disc heal. I instructed him to protect his disc and stay out of the crewing boat for a little while longer. I remember I looked at his mom and said, "With you or me it would have been twelve weeks before we got to this point. We would have needed epidurals, steroid shots, and everything else. Young people heal. Let's allow the natural healing course of his injury to continue. If he doesn't get back to 100 percent, I'll do prolotherapy to strengthen his back ligaments." Both Jeff and his mom were happy with this. If further problems arise for him, that would be the appropriate time for him to receive prolotherapy.

Timing of treatment is important. Like Jeff, a patient will occasionally come in too early and want to be aggressively treated. I tell him, "Let's give nature a chance to heal you. Eighty percent of the time, it will." Other patients come in too late and say, "I waited six months to see if I could heal myself." Often the injury has become chronic by the time they come to see me—which is not ideal. When it comes to starting treatment, it is better to err on the side of seeing your doctor early, to be sure of what the injury really is, and then letting him or her decide the right course of action.

ADDRESSING THE ISSUE

When I complete taking a patient's history and have done a thorough physical examination, I consider all the information I have gathered. I address what my patient thinks the issue might be, make my diagnosis, and explain to the patient what his options are. For example, if the patient has said, "Oh, I think my rotator cuff is torn," I might respond, "Well, I think your rotator cuff is fine, but you have some arthritis in your joint. Your history and physical are supporting that." This is a difficult conversation to initiate with a fifty-year-old who's been working out his whole life, playing sports his whole life, and then, seemingly all of a sudden, discovers he has this injury that is chronic or degenerative. Now, realistically, this "new-onset" arthritis has probably been brewing for twenty-five years but now, at age fifty, it has become symptomatic.

Such a discussion is very eye opening, and sobering for me as well as my patient. One of the tenets of sports medicine is, "Always try to keep the patient moving. Never tell them to stop." We pride ourselves in trying not to say to a patient, "Don't do that." But there comes a time, perhaps when a marathon runner has bone-on-bone arthritis of the hip, that his running days are coming quickly to an end. We have a "joke" in sports medicine— one designed to ease the blow. I'll say to the patient, "You know what we call a runner with arthritis of the hip?" And they say, "No, doc, what?" And they're very sincerely asking that question. I'll answer, "A cyclist." They realize that I'm trying to make it easier by telling a joke, and some chuckle. Then I say, "It's time to get ready to hang your running shoes up and pick another sport: something that's not going to be ground-pounding." I remind them that running imparts a gravitational impact on the weight-bearing joint that is three times that of walking and six times that of cycling.

Chas was such a patient. A marathon runner since high school, I discovered his knee arthritis had progressed to the bone-on-bone stage when he was fifty-seven. He had previously had episodic bouts of arthritis, and had treated them with the full spectrum of old-paradigm treatments, including numerous cortisone shots over the years. Before he came to me, he had gone to several orthopedic surgeons who told him it was time to stop running and get a double knee replacement. Chas was not ready to do that. He read about me online and came to see what a stem cell treatment could do to help. I told him there were no guarantees, but he was willing to give it a try.

However, I did tell him that he would need to find another sport, at least until we saw how well the treatment worked for him. At the time of writing, he was in the middle of the treatment regimen and was feeling a lot less pain, and increased mobility. At the proper time in between treatments, he was riding a mountain bike, sometimes for fairly long distances. Chas understood his body and knew for the stem cell injections to work, he would have to be very conscious of not stressing his knees too much. Will he be able to run in the future? Time will tell. However, he is happy being a cyclist for now and keeping his own knee joints.

A lot of times, patients aren't as cooperative as Chas. They are not ready to hear they need to change from a sport they love to one they don't. I really dislike delivering bad news, but it's my job at times to do so. I also realize patients hate to receive bad news. But in order to treat an injury in the proper way, there has to be an accurate diagnosis of what the issues are, a realization, and eventually an acceptance, that they might force you to make changes in your life.

WHAT YOU DO NOW CAN AFFECT YOU LATER

Medical awareness takes into account how much what you do now can affect your future. I recently treated a patient who ripped his meniscus apart and has arthritis. He said to me, "Doc, you've got to get me better so I can do this marathon, or so that I can play rugby or basketball in the over-fifty league." It seemed very important to him to keep his body going at a high level at this point in his life, even though it was falling apart before my eyes. I could temporarily get him back to that game, but is that in his best interest?

Martin was a businessman in his forties who lived to play racquetball. Whenever he had the opportunity, whether at home or traveling for business, he would be on the racquetball court. He came to see me when he hadn't been able to exercise for a year because it caused him severe pain. After thoroughly examining him and reading his x-rays, it was clear that he had bone-on-bone arthritis of the left hip. When I told him that, he was dumbfounded that it wasn't an acute injury that had been

---

I don't just want to keep people moving now: I want to keep them moving to their best capacity for the rest of their lives.

---

causing him his pain. He had a hard time believing that at his age, he could have such severe arthritis. We are going to try stem cell treatments on him because he is too young to get his joint replaced. Hopefully, through a course or two of stem cell treatments, we can hold off surgery for a number of years.

The more I practice medicine, the more I see patients in the baby boomer age group, like Martin. They are able to work or work out up to a point. Then an underlying problem, such as arthritis, kicks in, and they come to me, asking, "What happened to me? Why can't I move anymore?" I think a lot about the physician's responsibility to inform his patient of the risks of where he is headed. Recreational sport or repetitive, hard physical labor—especially as we age—gives doctors a never-ending supply of patients. I don't want to be that sports medicine guy who says, "You shouldn't be moving." However, I feel a patient needs to understand the future consequences of his current actions to decide whether he needs to make some changes in his occupational, fitness, sports or activity goals. I don't just want to keep people moving now: I want to keep them moving to their best capacity for the rest of their lives.

Maria was a house painter when she came to see me with an injury to her shoulder from falling off of a ladder. A former teacher, she liked painting more than teaching. She now owned her own company, and had for about ten years. When I examined her, I found a fairly severe tear in her rotator cuff, as well as mid-stage arthritis. Through PRP, I was able to help her mend the tear. However, I told Maria that if she kept painting, it was likely the repetitive motion would worsen her arthritis. Maria did not want to give up her business, so she was able to hire some younger people to do most of the actual painting, while she supervised and worked with clients. This, along with continuing RIT treatments, kept her arthritis from becoming severe.

When regenerative healing can slow the arthritic process down, as it did for Maria, it improves the quality of many people's lives. I am not saying these treatments are a cure for arthritis, because, at this time, they aren't yet. But used in a timely way, there is some good anecdotal evidence that prolotherapy, perineural superficial injections, PRP, and stem cell therapy all can greatly help early- and even mid-stage arthritis. It can also help those with more severe arthritis to delay joint replacement surgery. Since the expected life span of a replaced joint is ten to twenty years, delay is a very good thing. Boomers are the ones most likely to suffer from early arthritis now, but there is another trend that could make the onset of this disease even younger.

EARLY SPECIALIZATION

Earlier in the book, I expressed concern about the early sports specialization of young athletes. Of the over 600,000 youth baseball injuries treated by medical professionals every year, an increasing number are being treated with surgeries that were formerly reserved for older professional athletes seeking to prolong their careers. An example is the number of severe injuries to the ulnar collateral ligament of the elbow, which are increasingly being treated by a surgery called the "Tommy John" surgery.[1] At one prestigious sports medicine center, in the early 2000s, 18 percent of these surgeries were done on youth players; a decade later, the number of surgeries performed on young players had jumped to 31 percent.[2] Every time this topic comes up in medical meetings, there are bad statistics that go along with it.

Another extreme example of the problems of specialization is provided by a twelve-year-old who gets an anterior cruciate ligament (ACL) tear and has reconstructive surgery while he still has open growth plates. This makes the likelihood of him developing arthritis in his twenties pretty high, and the consequences of that will affect him for the rest of his life.

While some forms of RIT are appropriate for all ages, I prefer to reserve others, at this time, for my adult patients. However, other aspects of the new healing paradigm could definitely be used to cut down on the incidence of young patients undergoing musculoskeletal surgeries. This is particularly true because of the natural healing ability that most young people possess.

Utilizing the new healing paradigm with young athletes could offset some of the potential problems of this early sports specialization. Without such treatment, I am concerned that more patients could lose their functional mobility at an ever-younger age, which could lead to an arthritis nightmare for millions of patients. We could see a lot more formerly athletic people wheelchair-bound in the future after failing several joint replacement surgeries. It is important to remember that, until the late 1950s, when hip and knee replacements were developed, that was the eventual fate of anyone with severe arthritis.

EDGING TOWARD THE NEW

When my office was right across the hallway from the tennis barn at the Healthplex Sports Club, I had tennis player after tennis player coming in with tennis elbow. Martine was one of them. She told me, "I have had too many friends who failed physical therapy, had surgery, and became disaster cases. You've given me four steroid shots and a brace, and you've sent me to therapy three times. What else do you have? Because you've got to get me back to playing tennis—and I'm not getting surgery."

Before learning about RIT, I felt as though I was banging my head against the wall trying to help patients with this problem. After I was using the new paradigm, my fellows and I did a retrospective chart review on 125 patients suffering from tennis elbow who had come to see me. Two-thirds of them had a history of cortisone injections and said the cortisone helped, but only temporarily. All of them had failed other standard treatments for this injury: rest and physical therapy. About half of them had tried using a tennis elbow strap with the same poor results. They had exhausted the old-paradigm treatments for their injury. I had sent each patient to a type of myofascial release therapy called active release technique (ART), and about one-third required no further treatment. The other two thirds started receiving prolotherapy. These patients had a 90 percent cure rate. Of the 10 percent not cured, half of them reported improvement. This study period occurred before I brought diagnostic ultrasound to my practice. I believe the results could have been even more impressive with that tool. Shortly after my chart review, a controlled study by Drs. Michael Scarpone and David Rabago, et al., was published,[3] backing up my research and proving that prolotherapy was a very successful way to work with tennis elbow.

After an injury, if you don't heal within six weeks, you're falling into a chronic injury category, and with that diagnosis, many things can change in both your treatment and ultimate prognosis. It is critical that you use what you learn in this book to understand and recognize when you're not getting better as quickly as you should. Then start pursuing everything available to you in the new healing paradigm.

CHAPTER SEVEN
UNDERSTANDING PROLOTHERAPY

Nearly half of people with musculoskeletal problems have injuries stemming from tendons and ligaments rather than bones, joints, and muscles. Until the development of regenerative injection treatments (RIT), these patients had very few successful treatment options if they didn't heal on their own. If the old-paradigm standard of care of rest, physical therapy, anti-inflammatory medication, cortisone injections, bracing, ice, and manipulation didn't help their injury heal, they were left only with a surgical options. Successful surgery might be able to repair a patient's torn tendon or ligament, but it can also set the stage for or exacerbate arthritis, and a positive outcome is far from a guarantee. RIT bridges a critical gap in conventional treatments and offers hope to anyone suffering from a musculo-skeletal condition that previously had little chance for a cure.

Compared to surgery, RIT is relatively non-invasive and inexpensive. It can heal acute and chronic tendon, ligament, and cartilage injuries—torn meniscus, plantar fasciosis, carpal tunnel syndrome, and tennis elbow among others—as well as help arthritic joint pain and some other degenerative diseases.

Aside from perineural superficial injections (PSI), which stand in a class by themselves, prolotherapy is the simplest, least invasive, and least expensive of the four main regenerative injection treatments. Prolotherapy, platelet-rich plasma (PRP) injections, adult autologous stem cell (ASCI) injections, and PSI are all targeted biologic treatments. This means they are designed to help a patient's body heal itself.

With prolotherapy, lidocaine or procaine and dextrose or another proliferant solution are injected at the injured site. This stimulates the body's natural healing cascade. Essentially, these injections cause mild inflammation, drawing positive growth factors to the injured area. These begin to repair injured tissue, or improve the condition of a damaged joint, tendon, or ligament. The inflammation and any resulting pain are not treated using NSAIDs, like aspirin, ibuprofen, or naproxen, because, as I have detailed elsewhere, these commonly used medications can hamper the body's natural healing mechanisms. Following any initial discomfort, the patient can see and feel a positive difference, on average about a week or so after the injections.

HISTORY OF PROLOTHERAPY

Prolotherapy has been in use since the 1930s, when it was developed as a refinement of a treatment called sclerotherapy. Sclerotherapy is a non-surgical injection treatment developed in the mid-1800s to treat hemorrhoids and inguinal hernias. Sclerotherapy uses solutions which cause scarring fibrosis so veins can no longer fill up with blood and cause painful swelling. This seals the hernia pathways. Results were sufficiently satisfactory that sclerotherapy is still in use today. Now, it is used largely to treat varicose and other congested, poorly functioning veins.

The father of modern prolotherapy was a surgeon from Chicago, George Hackett, M.D., who, in the early 1950s, noticed there was apparently a similar scarring effect from the dextrose in the I.V. solutions used in hospitals. Any time he had to perform surgery on a patient, or do an autopsy on a deceased patient, Dr. Hackett would investigate this phenomenon. He would look for a residual scar from the I.V. dextrose. But rather than finding damage, he found evidence of healing, of stronger and more normal tissue where the I.V. solution had been. This inspired him to start using dextrose as a healing agent for damaged ligaments and tendons.

Dr. Hackett changed the name of the work he was doing from sclerotherapy to prolotherapy, from the Greek word *prolo* meaning "to grow," therefore, a therapy that creates new tissue. He also expanded using it only for tendon or ligament problems to using it inside the joint for arthritic conditions. In his later writings, he also acknowledged the link between the nerves in the fascia and the deeper tissues below, which eventually led to the development of PSI.

Dr. Hackett was way, way ahead of his time. He started teaching the methods he was using to some of his good friends and colleagues. One of them, Gustav Anders Hemwall, M.D., joined Dr. Hackett in his practice and helped form an early, core group of like-minded doctors. Dr. Hemwall and other physicians made service trips down to Central America to perform prolotherapy on poor, under-served patients, many of whom suffered both from severe, genetically caused varicose veins, and from a wide variety of musculoskeletal problems. Other doctors who wanted to learn how to perform this promising new treatment could come on these trips, help treat patients, and exchange ideas. This group of doctors eventually organized their work into the Hackett-Hemwall Foundation (HHF), now headed by one of my mentors in prolotherapy, Jeffery Patterson, D.O. The HHF has been traveling to Honduras for over forty years to train doctors from all over the world. For several years, after being trained in prolotherapy, I attended these service trips as a member of the teaching faculty. I have fond memories both of the rewarding work we did and of the friends I made.

Other doctors, some of them very well-known, have been interested in prolotherapy, and have provided considerable support for this work. President John F. Kennedy's personal physician was a woman named Janet Travell, M.D. She, along with David G. Simons, M.D., authored *Myofascial Pain and Dysfunction: The Trigger Point Manual.*[1] While her work was groundbreaking, she still felt it merely scratched the surface of what could be ultimately possible. It is said that on Dr. Travell's deathbed, she urged one of her junior students, George Yu, M.D., a rising star urologic surgeon, to find the link between trigger point therapy and prolotherapy. Dr. Yu, who was granted a teaching fellowship at the National Institute of Health (NIH), was able to help get some of the research about prolotherapy funded by the NIH.

Prolotherapy works by triggering the immune system's healing cascade.

C. Everett Koop, M.D., former Surgeon General of the United States, was also a proponent of prolotherapy. I have heard his story was similar to mine. He was unable to work as a pediatric general surgeon without experiencing severe pain, and was considering going on disability. He had several prolotherapy treatments, which gave him so much relief he was able to continue working. Then he learned how to do prolotherapy himself and treated friends and family members. Since he was a pediatrician, he did not use it on his patients. At that time, it was not known how younger patients would respond to prolotherapy. But he did treat his patient's parents when they complained to him about their musculoskeletal pain.

There are reports of letters written by Dr. Koop indicating he was in a letter-writing battle with Medicare trying to get prolotherapy approved. At that time, there was little literature, and only some very poorly done research showing that prolotherapy worked. Today there is a lot more research and literature of excellent quality. Yet the naysayers at Medicare still are saying the same thing they did earlier: there isn't enough research to enable them to approve prolotherapy.

HOW PROLOTHERAPY WORKS

Prolotherapy has been, and continues to be employed by cutting-edge physicians to tighten and strengthen weak and damaged ligaments and tendons, which otherwise cause both pain and instability. It is also used to decrease pain and improve function in some forms of arthritis and nerve damage. The technique requires the injection of a local anesthetic (procaine or lidocaine) to numb the area plus 10 to 25 percent dextrose (a form of sugar), and, if needed to stimulate a stronger healing response, the addition of sodium morrhuate (highly refined cod liver oil) or other less commonly used proliferant solutions. The injection is made at the point where the ligament or tendon attaches to the bone, at the joint capsule, inside the joint, or in the myofascial layer. I have read estimates that the procedure has been used on well over one million patients and has been proven as safe as other types of injections commonly used in orthopedics.[2]

Prolotherapy works by triggering the immune system's healing cascade. Following an injury, your body releases prostaglandin, causing inflammation, which attracts white blood cells, other immune system cells and platelets. This causes the release of various growth factors, which can repair or improve the damaged tissue. Remember, any discomfort caused by the injection is not treated using NSAIDs, which are prostaglandin inhibitors. If you sprain your ankle and it becomes very painful, swollen, red, warm to the touch, that's prostaglandin at work. If you inhibit prostaglandin in the early healing phase of an injury, you limit the "stage" for the remodeling that can occur in that ligament. The larger the healing stage, the greater the potential for a completely healed ligament.

Prolotherapy's local inflammatory reaction begins this tissue repair process. It is normal and expected to experience some pain at the injection site for a few days. It is common after injections to have some swelling, particularly when the injection has been in the extremities. People have a wide range of responses to prolotherapy, from some who have virtually no discomfort to others who suffer an excessive or super-inflammatory response, where the inflammation doesn't calm down for several days, but instead can take one to three weeks. If the discomfort is too great, it is treated with a non-NSAID pain medication and/or ice.

HEALING TAKES TIME

A single prolotherapy treatment sets the healing stage, but the healing process—just as it is with surgery—is lengthy and gradual. Surgeons used to be very quick to get a professional athlete back to the field of play after reconstruction of a ligament. Now they know patients don't do as well when they are rushed back to play in three or four months. Today, they try to have them end their season after the injury, get reconstructed, and then not return to play for at least nine to twelve months. The athletes can work out, they can do physical therapy and start doing hard training at four to six months, but they are not expected to go back to the same

When you treat a ligament with prolotherapy, it kicks in a natural healing process that lasts about 100 days.

level of play until about a year after the reconstruction. That's all about healing properly, which takes time. For example, when I had PRP in my shoulder, four weeks later, I was unhappy I did the treatment; six weeks later, I was back to baseline; and eight weeks later, I felt so much better I was glad I did the treatment. I continued to notice improvement throughout the year.

I know this sounds strange, but when you treat a ligament with prolotherapy, it kicks in a natural healing process that lasts about one hundred days. The patient's body initially has an inflammatory reaction, which lasts approximately four days. The healing process then moves into the granulation phase where fibroblast cells begin to lay down new collagen, one of the main building blocks of our connective tissue. These cells begin to prepare the body for the third and final healing stage, remodeling. The reason why someone continues to get better after a single treatment is that remodeling takes many months. The bulk of it is done in one to three months, but it will continue on for the rest of that year. A patient who's had numerous prolotherapy treatments could continue this healing process long after his treatments ceased. Melanie is an example.

As a young girl, Melanie loved riding horses. Of course, she had many spills, and, like most children thirty years ago, she received little treatment for them. She grew up to be a realtor, whose hobby was "flipping houses." She and a partner bought shells of homes in Philadelphia, demolished and then rebuilt them. During one of her renovations, she started having back pain, which got worse over time. Over the years Melanie tried everything, except surgery. She had eight years of constant acupuncture, which temporarily alleviated but did not cure the pain. She went to chiropractors. She went to doctors who gave her steroid injections and prescribed physical therapy.

"You name it," Melanie said, "if it is out there I tried it. I was begging for anything that would put me out of my misery, but nothing was helping. I was in pain 24/7; it was just a question

---

> "For the next twelve years, I just gritted my teeth and ran. My Achilles pain was always there, ranging between four and five on the pain scale."

---

of how much. The center of the excruciating pain was my lower back. I saw neurosurgeons, orthopedic surgeons, the whole gamut. In 2003, I was bed-ridden for three months. My back problems continued for twenty years." Then a distant cousin heard about my practice from his physician, and he told Melanie. By the time I saw her, she had several herniated discs, annular tears, spinal stenosis, and total dehydration of the disc at one level.

When she began the prolotherapy treatments she continued every six weeks for two years. Melanie described her process as "a long, hard climb," but one in which she was showing incremental improvement. She reported every treatment was different. The healing process this therapy initiates continues over many weeks and months. Thus, the most substantial improvement in her condition happened over the course of the year in which she had to relocate and suspend treatments. Melanie said at that time she practically felt like she had a new back and could do almost everything. "I am fully functional now whereas I was barely functional before. Now I'm at a zero pain level most of the time."

DON'T GIVE UP

Anthony is a financial planner who has always been very active in his time off. He played baseball, softball, and tennis before discovering running, which has been his passion for thirty years. He would run forty-five to fifty miles a week, had participated in several marathons, and was in training for another distance run when he felt a slight hamstring pull while playing softball. When the pain passed, he returned to running as though he had not missed a day. Within a month, he felt a problem in his left Achilles tendon that he had never noticed before. When he would run for a mile or two, the pain would go away. Consequently, he kept running up to fifty miles a week for fifteen months, until he got to the point when he couldn't run anymore. He went to an orthopedic sports medicine doctor, who gave him cortisone shots and a heel lift and told him to stop running until his pain subsided.

"I didn't run for four months, which was an eternity for me."

So, he told me, he began to run again and just put up with the pain. "For the next twelve years, I just gritted my teeth and ran. My Achilles pain was always there, ranging between four and five on the pain scale. One year, I ran 130 road races. In 2007, a friend told me about you. At that point, my pain was constantly about seven."

I examined Anthony and discussed prolotherapy with him. Although it was the first time he had heard of it, he was willing to give it a try. I sent him for MRIs and x-rays, and found Achilles tendinosis, with a bone spur also contributing to his pain. I began

"To me, my healing is miraculous."

prolotherapy treatments and continued them every six to eight weeks for more than ten treatments. I also had to remove his bone spur with a large needle several times to help him eventually heal. I encouraged Anthony not to run for seven to ten days after each treatment when I removed the bone spur and five days if I solely did prolotherapy. As the treatments continued, he experienced less and less pain, and by the end of two years, his tendon was 100 percent healed. I later treated him for shin splints and a torn hamstring. By that time, I was also using PRP and ASCI in my practice, but Anthony preferred that I keep treating him with prolotherapy, and it worked for him every time.

"It took two years to heal my Achilles injury, but if you talk to other runners with long-term Achilles problems, they will tell you it never goes away. I feared that would be my situation until I came to you. To me, my healing is miraculous. I would urge other runners not to give up. There is help out there, if you are willing to look for it."

A DIFFICULT CASE SUCCEEDS

Gary is a contractor who finished having prolotherapy treatment five years before being interviewed for this book. He has never since that time had a recurrence of the extreme pain in his feet that originally brought him to me.

Recalling his earlier problems, Gary said, "I suddenly started getting such bad pain in my feet that I could barely walk. I woke up in the morning with throbbing feet, and the pain would radiate into my calves and my back. I could not walk for more than fifteen minutes without being in intolerable pain. For over a year, I went to every kind of doctor I could find. They gave me multiple diagnoses, and nearly every one of them had me in a wheelchair. I was in a terrible situation." Gary talked again to his family doctor who, by then, had heard of my work. She suggested Gary see me. I found chronic plantar fasciosis, sprained ligaments, and an extremely high instep in Gary's feet. Gary was surprised when I told him what he had could be dealt with and, in all likelihood, cured. I originally anticipated doing three or four treatments, but, as it turned out, Gary was "super inflammatory." He experienced little initial pain from the shots, but at about the second week, the treatments would cripple him for several weeks. This was not a good thing for a contractor who needed to be mobile.

Most patients under a doctor's care let the physician take charge and lay out the game plan. Not so with Gary. He listened to me, but he would say, "You know, I noticed that my pain relief didn't start until right around the time that you were getting ready to treat me again, so how about if instead of coming back in four weeks, I come back in eight weeks and see how good I get?" We agreed to try this and eventually figured out Gary didn't need to be treated every four weeks: An eight-week frequency seemed to work best for him. The first week after treatment he'd feel reasonably good, and then he would have fairly severe pain for a few weeks. When it calmed down, he would feel a lot of improvement. Gary reported, "It just devastated me when I got it done, but each time I improved a little bit." By the time we came to the middle of Gary's treatments, he was seeing a significant turnaround and was very happy. Toward the end of his treatments, the process was less painful and his healing time quicker. It took him about ten treatments to get better, but we did get him better. Before, he had been crippled and looking at disability.

"Prolotherapy works. I'm cured and have been fine for over five years. I've learned not to overdo it, and to always wear the proper shoes and orthotics," Gary said enthusiastically. "I owe my ability to walk to you and prolotherapy."

FROM GYMNASTICS TO DIVING, THROUGH PROLOTHERAPY

Brittany began gymnastics when she was three years old. Like many serious gymnasts, she had a lot of injuries along the way. When she was ten, she broke the fifth metatarsal bone in her foot and was put in a hard cast. Following her recovery from that, she experienced a shoulder injury that kept her out of gymnastics for a full year. She then broke her hand and was put in a cast for that. She had to wear a brace for cartilage that was loose in her knee. She sprained her ankles multiple times.

However, it was her back injuries that really caused her distress. The problems started with pain in her sacroiliac joints and with sacrotuberous ligament problems. Despite all this, she kept performing as a gymnast until she fractured the fifth lumbar vertebra of her spine when she was in high school. The doctor she was seeing tried burning the nerves around the joint, then gave her nerve block injections. She tried acupuncture for pain relief. She was braced four times and had used an electronic bone stimulator. When all of these failed to give her relief, she went to see an osteopathic physician in another state who specialized in working with gymnasts headed for the Olympics. He worked on her

---

"I owe my ability to walk to you and prolotherapy."

---

using osteopathic manipulation and was able to relieve her pain. But the alignment would not hold. Her orthopedic surgeons told her she would not get relief from the pain unless they fused the fractures. She and her parents finally agreed to the surgery. After recovering from the spinal fusion, she started doing gymnastics again until she fractured her back once more and also injured a disc. She was put in a back brace for four months. During that time, a doctor mentioned prolotherapy. She and her parents had a difficult time finding someone who practiced this form of treatment. She was originally referred to a doctor in Connecticut, but since she lived in Maryland, that physician referred her to me. She first saw me about a year and a half after she had the spinal fusion, when she was nineteen years old.

Over a nine-month period I worked on her entire back. Since she was attending a college in the Midwest, she flew in to the Philadelphia area on a Friday morning, met her parents at the airport, got her prolotherapy treatment in my office, and flew back to school on Sunday. At first I was treating her on a monthly basis, but then I started to space out the treatments to see how well her back held. After her first prolotherapy treatment, she felt good enough to begin diving for her college at a Division I level. As things continued to hold, I gave her a six-month break. After that she only needed a yearly "tune-up."

Brittany reported, "Prolotherapy has helped me so much. I don't regret having surgery because I know I had other issues, but I wish I had looked into prolotherapy more before the surgery. I don't think prolo affected the surgical sites but it helped everything around them. Even if I had not had the surgery, it still might have worked. It has helped me immensely . . . after every treatment I felt better."

EVERYTHING HAS IMPROVED

Kevin went into the Marine Corps directly after college. He quickly rose through the ranks to become a captain. A high school athlete, he was very physically fit and enjoyed the challenges of Marine life. When he was twenty-nine, during a military training exercise he was directing, he became injured with what was diagnosed as a herniated disc in his spine. He kept up his physical pace despite the pain. The injury became worse. It got to the point where he couldn't sit for more than ten minutes, or drive a car. The doctors determined he had another herniation, compressed against a nerve.

Kevin was told his only option was to have an operation to relieve the pressure. In a study at a prestigious university, he was case 109 of 111 and the only one who failed back surgery, meaning he was in worse shape after the operation than before. Nonetheless, he proceeded to physical therapy, which got him back on his feet, but gave him a number of other problems, including completely unpredictable pain and numbness that would travel down his left leg. It turned out that in physical therapy he had ruptured the two discs on top of the previously herniated ones. He was in his early thirties and parts of his spine were beginning to collapse. Kevin was told that before he was thirty-five he was going to need to have his spine surgically fused.

Kevin had heard of me through his wife and some friends, but only became a patient after seeing me appear on ESPN's SportsCenter. I suggested an initial prolotherapy protocol of six to ten sessions. After the tenth treatment, Kevin was only getting about ten days of relief following each session. I felt this wasn't a good enough outcome to continue, so I discussed stopping prolotherapy. But after that treatment, Kevin had a breakthrough and enjoyed three weeks of relief. Because of that, he and I agreed to continue with the prolotherapy, but we allowed him to rest about two months between treatments.

"Where I was to where I am now is night and day," Kevin said. "Am I perfect? No. But the other side of the coin is that I still have 90 percent range of motion. Prolotherapy wasn't the 100 percent answer for me; maybe only 75 percent. But that 75 percent is a lot better than any other recommendations I got from health care. My quality of life, my work as a schoolteacher, my relationship with my wife and family, everything improved since I started seeing you."

Besides offering him some relief with the prolotherapy treatments, Kevin reported, "You were also the first doctor to look at my blood work, telling me that when you have chronic pain, the adrenal gland is often overworked. This upsets the entire system, making your hormones go way off and affecting your mood. You were the first doctor to make me aware of that connection, and that awareness helped me greatly in my healing."

BACK IN THE GAME

My youngest prolotherapy patient to date was Richard, then a nine-year-old boy whose mother I had treated with prolotherapy for a knee injury. The mother came to me in tears because something had happened to Richard's thumb and he could barely move it. Upon examination, I concluded he had sprained his ulnar collateral ligament and sent Richard to a surgeon to be evaluated for reconstructive surgery. The surgeon said he could not help Richard until the boy finished growing because he had open growth plates. The doc would need to drill through the growth plate to reconstruct the ligament. The mother came back to me even more upset and asked me if there was anything I could do. She explained that her son could no longer play ball with his friends or play the trombone, two activities he really enjoyed. It was even difficult for Richard to write notes in classes or to do his homework. She reported that some of his friends would no longer play with him because he couldn't hold or throw a ball. Although I do not like to offer prolotherapy to children as a treatment, I agreed because it seemed to be the only option the boy had left.

After two treatments, Richard came back with a ball in his hand and a smile on his face. I told him, "Throw me the ball." After Richard threw it, I threw it back and he caught it barehanded. I checked him out and told him he was done and should go play with his friends.

Eight years later the same mother returned with her daughter with a fractured wrist. She told me that Richard, now seventeen years old, was enjoying a full high school career with a lot of sports activity, and that his thumb had never bothered him again.

A GORGEOUS TENDON

One of my older prolotherapy patients had a truly surprising outcome to her treatments. When I met Cora ten years ago, she was in her mid-sixties. I really didn't think she was a very good candidate for the treatment because of her age and because she was a smoker who just didn't take good care of herself. Cora had been injured when she slipped and fell in a casino, tearing her rotator cuff pretty badly and severely hurting her lower back. She was represented by a lawyer because of this incident. Research has shown that in a litigation situation, a patient is less likely to get well.[3] I was willing to treat Cora, but because of her legal situation, along with her general poor health, I did not know how successful the treatment would be.

When Cora first came in, she was really just begging for help because no one else had given her any hope they could effectively treat her. The other doctors she had seen had told her she was not a good surgical candidate, and she was just going to have to live with her condition. She had received a couple of steroid shots, but these hadn't worked, and Cora was miserable.

I told her, "We'll have to alternate your treatments: I will treat your back one session and I'll do your shoulder the next. These are going to be big treatments which are going to hurt and will require recovery time. I don't want to cripple you by treating both areas at once." She understood, and we started. I treated Cora five times in the shoulder and four times in the lower back. Each time she came in, she commented on what she'd experienced. She noticed how the treatments were helping her, and how she could move her arm more. She was starting to get more and more excited. When she came in for her next scheduled shoulder treatment, she said, "Doc, I don't need any more treatments. I'm better."

I had treated her using a diagnostic ultrasound machine for guidance, and I have before and after pictures showing her rotator cuff. After those treatments, her tendon looked like that of a twenty-five-year-old. It's gorgeous. I wrote to some of my colleagues and said, "You're not going to believe this. We always talk about how we can treat patients with prolotherapy, but we don't often think about the treatment as potentially helpful for a very injured and poor-healing potential patient who is a smoker in her upper years. We don't think about prolotherapy returning the tissues of such a patient back to normal. We think we can treat

---

"I look forward to walking in, treating my patients, and getting them better. That's what gets me up in the morning."

---

their pain and maybe get some healing, but we're not taught that the tissue could be normal again after we're done treating them. Well, look at this case!"

A number of years later, Cora fell again, this time at her home. She sustained a nasty leg fracture, which required surgical insertion of plates and screws to secure it. One of the screws went right through her bone and was irritating a nerve next to the bone. She had nerve pain from her toes to her outer thigh. I did two PSI treatments, a hydrodissection of a superficial nerve, and two prolotherapy treatments to a torn tendon and torn ankle ligament. Six weeks later, Cora came back and reported that she felt cured.

When I use diagnostic ultrasound to look at my patients' injured tissue and guide the needle to the exact target, it's exciting to look back over the images to see their progress over time. Cora's case is but one example. It's clear that there is an excellent potential in most patients to heal. If we put the needle in the right place with the right solution in the right amount with the right frequency, and we give the patient proper education on how to take care of his diseased joint, tendon, or ligament, he has a strong possibility of healing. I see it every day in my practice. It always amazes me when I can take what looks like a tendon that's been hit by a grenade and, through RIT, see it return to normal. I look forward to walking in, treating my patients, and getting them better. That's what gets me up in the morning.

There have been cases so severe that I've been skeptical whether even RIT could help. Usually the patient is desperate and almost begs me to give it a try. When I do, over 50 percent of the time, even in those severe cases, prolotherapy makes a big difference. Prolo works. If it doesn't give patients all of the relief they are looking for, then we can go to PRP or ASCI. But I like to start with prolotherapy whenever it is medically advisable. It is less expensive and requires less downtime post treatment.

PROLOTHERAPY AS PANACEA

Prolotherapy is finally becoming popularized, and now some orthopedic surgeons are incorporating it into their practices. I see this as a big positive—so long as the surgeon has the training and expertise to do it, and is willing to take the time to perform the treatments properly. However, some practices are doing prolotherapy in the orthopedic model, and that just does not work. I'm hearing of instances of quick, joint-specific evaluations and maybe a single injection. In an orthopedic practice, many times the patient's evaluation by the doctor takes five minutes. For prolotherapy to work, the doctor cannot focus only on the area of pain. He must look at least at the joint above and the joint below, look at the stabilizing ligaments around the joint and the joint capsule. He should also see how the patient walks and stands, and dynamically assess the joint.

I had a patient recently, Evelyn, who had gone to a doctor who was one of the fellows I had trained in sports medicine. She said the doctor spent five minutes with her, and within those five minutes, he was offering her prolotherapy to her spine. He never laid hands on her, never looked at any films. I'm sure he's in a very busy practice, and has been trained in that setting to do things that way, but from his training with me, he should know better.

Evelyn said, "I didn't know what prolotherapy was. I was very fearful and anxious. I wanted to get out of there. I would never go back to a doctor who just, literally within a few minutes of meeting me, was offering to put needles in my back." After the forty minutes I spent with her, she felt very comfortable with my treatment plan, and it all made sense to her. I am not going to offer her prolotherapy unless she fails physical therapy. She's going to get films, I'm going to assess them and make an accurate diagnosis, and lay out a treatment plan that makes sense. If Evelyn fails a comprehensive, conservative plan, then we'll talk about prolotherapy more seriously down the road.

That orthopedic practice specifically hired two of the sports medicine fellows I had trained, knowing I had taught them prolotherapy. They wanted to bring prolotherapy to their practice, but they're doing it in the orthopedic model. This is where the surgeon walks in the room, says, "Hi, how you doing? Do you need surgery or not? Do you need prolotherapy first?" The doctor answers that question within five minutes, and out he goes. That's what that doctor was trying to do with Evelyn. It just doesn't work that way. Prolotherapy is not a panacea. For many people it can be a miraculous healing treatment method, but only if it is practiced in the proper way, which takes time and expertise.

CHAPTER EIGHT
UNDERSTANDING PERINEURAL SUPERFICIAL INJECTIONS AND BIOPUNCTURE

Prolotherapy is based on the use of hypertonic dextrose (or sugar water) injected into joints, ligaments, tendons, and muscles. It causes a growth factor increase in the injured tissue and begins a natural healing process lasting long after the treatment has ceased. Perineural superficial injections (PSI) have also been called neural-fascial injection treatments (NFIT), superficial perineural injections (SPNI), and superficial (or neural) prolotherapy. This technique, developed by John Lyftogt, M.D., in New Zealand in the early twenty-first century,[1] consists of injections of low-dose (5 percent) dextrose or dextrose with a small amount of lidocaine (or now other agents, like mannitol or glycerin) administered near the nerves that lie just beneath the skin. The injection is performed with a small needle that is placed right under the skin. Other than local injection site soreness or a small bruise, adverse effects are uncommon.

PSI reduces or eliminates superficial nerve pain from a neuropathic pain source. It does not specifically work to heal injured joints, ligaments, tendons, and muscles, although it can have a helpful effect on healing in those structures in some cases. Because of this treatment's anti-inflammatory effect on the nerves, it allows them to return to their normal, healthy state within six to eight treatments. There is proof that 5 percent dextrose reduces the output of specific nerve protein molecules called neuropeptides, which are released by the inflamed, swollen nerve.[2] Low-dose dextrose can break this cycle, most likely because it

---

> Because of this treatment's anti-inflammatory effect on the nerves, it allows them to return to their normal, healthy state within six to eight treatments.

---

binds to presynaptic calcium channels and stops the body from releasing substance P, nitrous oxide, and calcitonin gene-related peptide (CGRP), all of which increases inflammation of these superficial nerves. Without this, the swollen nerve is caught in a vicious cycle. PSI can break the cycle and allow the nerve to recover. It can offer a success rate of greater than 75–80 percent for chronic neuropathic pain conditions that previously had few effective treatments.

The low-dose dextrose in PSI blocks calcium, thus breaking the aforementioned inflammatory cycle. In classic prolotherapy, the dextrose injection mimics an injury and initiates the healing cascade. While this cascade causes initial inflammation and swelling, it also gives the body a push to naturally heal the injury. I've been using PSI since it was first introduced by Dr. Lyftogt to U.S. physicians at the University of Wisconsin in Madison in 2006. Because the treatment is so new, it is still a work in progress, with physicians frequently finding new ways to use it. Already, there has been a well-designed, randomized controlled trial showing this treatment to be superior to standard treatment for Achilles tendinosis.[3] Most of Dr. Lyftogt's patients reported that the 5 percent dextrose solution relieved pain in the area within minutes of administration,[4] with the pain decrease lasting up to five days. I have found that adding a tiny amount of lidocaine to the dextrose solution assures a more comfortable experience for all my patients. A little lidocaine also gives an immediate numbing block to help me decide if this treatment will be effective for a patient. When you put dextrose around a nerve, it only numbs an area the size of a dime. When you put lidocaine around a nerve, the numbing area is larger and lasts for at least an hour. So when the patient gets up and starts moving around, he feels really numb, and when that lidocaine-induced numbness wears off, the dextrose is working. Most of the time the pain relief lasts for quite a while. Typically, patients require six to eight treatments, done weekly or every two weeks. Most patients report 10–15 percent improvement per week.

My patient Helena was very grateful for that initial pain relief, since she had suffered from constant chronic pain for almost four years before treatment. She had been in a bad auto accident when she was in her twenties, almost twenty years before. A lively woman, Helena had been working for a pharmaceutical company doing training, a job that required a lot of travel. She kept working as much as possible throughout her post-accident years. Because her professional background was in mainstream medicine, she did not know she had any alternatives.

Helena sought out the best of old-paradigm care for her injured neck, shoulder, and back. She had received over two dozen procedures—such as epidurals, nerve testing, blocks—and six surgeries before I saw her. Her spine was fused from her neck to her waist. She contracted a post-operative wound infection, which required yet another surgery. She had a lot of scar tissue that almost felt like rope in various parts of her body. Because of the pain from her scar tissue and other injuries, Helena was suffering from chronic regional pain syndrome (CRPS) type 1. Doctors often misdiagnose this condition, as they did in her case, as fibromyalgia. A tenacious woman who was determined to function as well as possible, Helena eventually found out about and tried myofascial release work and chiropractic manipulation. She reported they both helped, but she still had extreme leg pain and found it difficult to sit for any period of time.

"Eventually my chiropractor recommended I see you," she told me, adding that she was willing to do whatever she had to in order to heal. Because of prolonged chronic pain affecting many parts of her body, I decided to begin with PSI to try to calm down the pain. I literally treated her from her neck to her low back. I saw her weekly for four months, and she reported a significant pain decrease, estimating she was about 40 percent better.

When she was up to it, I began to add classic prolotherapy to treat her ligaments and affected facet joints. Later, I added work on her stellate and sympathetic ganglions. These are a collection of nerves in the neck and lower back, and I find nerve blocks in this area useful for people, like Helena, who have had prolonged pain or major trauma. She reported these injections helped her psychologically as well as physically.

"I am always still in pain," she reported, "but it is at least 75 percent less pain than I had when I began seeing you about eighteen months ago. That is amazing, because I have had about a

70 percent improvement in my functioning while the pain has decreased. I am able to travel a lot for business. I have learned that traditional medicine does not have all the answers. I think it is unfortunate that not everyone knows there are these other options. I also think it is too bad that insurance does not cover it. This makes it less accessible to a lot of people who would be helped by it. I also respect that you take seriously your Hippocratic Oath to do no harm. Because these methods are so powerful, they must be done with due care, and you are sure to take that care."

CRPS, type 1, is a very difficult diagnosis to treat and manage. If a patient comes to me with this diagnosis, and I am able to pinpoint the primary cause of the CRPS, then I might be able to help it using new-paradigm treatments. Unfortunately, we still don't have a good answer about what causes this type of pain, and so I have only had success treating it in some cases.

HOW PSI WORKS

Perineural superficial injections work on the nerves that travel under our skin and provide sensation to it. Superficial nerves include nerves with and without myelin. Pain-sensing nerves do not have myelin, the substance that protects and speeds up impulses in some other nerves in the body. These branch out from deeper nerves that provide sensation at the spinal-cord level. They supply sensation to blood vessels, nerves, muscles, ligaments, tendons, bone, joint capsules, and cartilage. This treatment can affect a patient's pain because superficial and deep nerves are connected. Every superficial nerve crossing a joint has branches that innervate the joint itself. Injecting dextrose, an analgesic and anti-inflammatory agent, around inflamed, swollen superficial nerves can calm down the inflammation that is causing the nerve to swell. This allows the nerve to shrink and stops the entrapment between the nerve and myofascial connective tissue. Normal nerve function going upstream and downstream from the point of injection is restored, along with the release of regenerative growth factors, which may help maintain tissue health at the end of the nerve.

PSI can be used before other RIT treatments, since entrapped nerves can often prevent underlying musculoskeletal problems from healing, which prevents other RIT treatments from working as well as possible. PSI also can be used to give pain relief in between other treatments. For example, in half of my cases of chronic disc problems in the lower back that have not resolved with the usual treatments, the addition of PSI injections has helped to treat the underlying nerve inflammation.[5]

Let's consider the case of my elbow. I have a torn tendon in my elbow, and I keep aggravating it because every week I'm doing too much around my house or straining the tendon while treating my patients. My healing takes two steps forward and one step back. When my torn tendon is aggravated, the nerves around my elbow and down my forearm are more painful. I can feel the tender, swollen nerves running over my elbow, next to my tendon. When my tendon is feeling better, the same nerves feel better and shrink in size. So, when will my forearm stop hurting? That will happen when the tendon is healed. I have tried PSI as a standalone treatment for my elbow injury, and it has given me temporary pain relief, but every time I look at my injury with ultrasound, the injury is unchanged. What I'm finding in my practice is, if I pay attention to the nerves with PSI and also go after the deep tissue damage with classic prolotherapy, PRP, and ASCI, I see the best results. Until I see good Level I evidence that I can heal everything that I'm treating with PRP, stem cells, and prolotherapy with PSI, I am going to continue using whichever combination of treatments can bring the most pain relief and healing to my patients.

For PSI to be most effective, it needs to be repeated before the effect wears off and swelling recurs. If not repeated within a few weeks, the swelling and inflammation will return, and the nerve improvement will be lost. On the average, repeating the treatment six to eight times at weekly or biweekly intervals will allow the swollen nerve to return to normal function. Then the healing powers of the body will take over, and, in many cases, the nerve will stay normal and stop transmitting pain permanently.

Because PSI produces a reduction in pain almost immediately, there is no downtime following this treatment, nor is rehabilitation necessary. In most people, the PSI injections continue working for five to seven days, although with succeeding treatments, the effects tend to last longer. I have had some patients report that their pain went away with only one treatment, but more commonly the patient starts to notice lasting pain relief after a series of six to eight treatments. As healing sets in, the size of the area I need to treat also decreases.

EFFECTIVE USE OF PSI

I wouldn't think of using PSI if a patient doesn't have superficial pain. There are some cases where PSI does help a deeper structure heal, but in many cases, its effectiveness is limited to nerve pain or neuropathic pain relief.

I treated Terry, a patient whose Achilles tendon was partially torn. His chronically diseased tendon had abnormal calcification throughout it. Terry had been suffering for about a year and had gone through various old-paradigm treatments. I palpated his leg upstream from his tendon, where we typically find the superficial nerves in the calf are inflamed. Terry didn't even know he had pain up there, which is not unusual when pain in one area is particularly severe. As I started palpating these nerves in his calf, Terry was dancing all over the table trying to get away from my thumbs. He said, "I had no idea it even hurt up there." Terry's case is a perfect example of how the nerves are linked and associated with his chronic injury down in his Achilles tendon. With Terry, it was not enough for me to only treat the tendon. I treated his nerves with PSI four times before he came back for his PRP. His Achilles tendon healed up with eight PSI treatments and two PRP treatments. Before using this combination treatment, it would have taken at least four PRP treatments to get a similar outcome.

Cindy was a different matter. She had pain in her Achilles tendon area. I looked with my ultrasound and it looked perfect. There was no abnormality. The tendon was normal size, and there were no features on ultrasound or on MRI that showed Cindy's tendons were diseased. I examined the nerves in her calf and found them to be extremely irritated. Cindy would not need any formal prolotherapy or PRP into the tendon; I would only need to treat her nerves.

A third patient, Selena, comes in with the same problem. She's tender only over the tendon. I palpated her calf where all the nerve branches are, and I could find nothing. Since she did not present any of the signs of superficial nerve pain, I did not offer her PSI. I would only offer her injections directly into the diseased tendon with prolotherapy, or, if necessary, PRP.

I see a mix of several types of patients out there: ones who have primary disease in the deeper structure, ones with only nerves involved, and ones who have problems with both. An important part of the physical exam is assessing whether a particular patient has these inflamed nerves radiating to a superficial level, or whether his injury is isolated to the deeper structure. There is no clear-cut answer to the question, "When are perineural superficial injections the slam dunk treatment of choice?" I would certainly consider it for Achilles tendon issues, anterior knee pain problems, low back pain, rib pain in the thorax, any scar pain or radiating pain that has been ruled in or out for a herniated disc, frozen shoulder, tennis and golfer's elbow, chronic hamstring injuries, nerve entrapment by surgical hardware, chronic exertional compartment syndrome, some kinds of headaches, and other neck or head injuries.

PSI AND FROZEN SHOULDER

I treated Candice, a woman in her early forties, who came in with a socked-in frozen shoulder. She believed the reason her shoulder went bad was because she had taken an antibiotic in the fluoroquinalone family of drugs. Evidently, this reaction is common enough that at least one website has been launched to serve the affected community.[6] People who post on the site call it being "floxed." Candice and her online friends believe in a medical theory with limited evidence, which has indicated the fluoroquinalone antibiotic family only affects a small percentage of the population. These people likely possess a defect in their mitochondrial systems that causes sensitivity to these drugs. People subscribing to this theory contend that this defect is insignificant until people with this sensitivity take fluoroquinalones. Then, they believe, this drug class poisons such people's nerves, and it is unlikely such people will ever be normal again.

In an earlier chapter, I recounted other reports of ciprofloxen damaging ligaments and tendons, so I believe some of these concerns may be founded in fact. In our initial interview, Candice told me she had taken three consecutive courses of a fluoroquinalone antibiotic for a suspected sinus infection, which turned out to be caused by an allergy to her sleep apnea equipment. She reported she was healthy up until this infection, but shortly after began to experience some strange reactions. When she injured her Achilles tendon putting on a shoe, she knew she needed help. She went to a well-respected orthopedic clinic but received little relief. She also said the clinician was skeptical that her tendon problems were connected with the drug.

She began to develop shoulder pain. She went to another orthopedic practice and was put on aggressive physical therapy. Candice told me that only aggravated the pain and stiffness in her shoulder. She then sought help from an integrative medicine practice because she was experiencing worsening physical and emotional effects. There she was treated with intravenous nutrition, which helped many of her physical and emotional symptoms. However, her shoulder pain was still worsening. The integrative doctor referred her to me.

When I first saw her, she had one of the worst frozen shoulders I had ever seen. Before PSI, I would refer a patient like this to surgery for manipulation under general anesthesia. My experience with such severely frozen shoulders had demonstrated to me that it would be too painful to even try a new-paradigm RIT procedure. PSI appears to work on a frozen shoulder by calming down the nerves around the shoulder. This also relieves pain in the affected, overly tight muscles and fascia that cause the loss of range of motion. I explained to Candice that first I had to calm down her nerve pain because her nerves were excessively inflamed and swollen.

In my first session with her, I administered over one hundred PSI injections in her arm, shoulder, chest, and neck. She told me she experienced no miraculous cure, but that she could feel a difference in a few days. Her shoulder was less stiff. Using ultrasound diagnosis, I also found a tear, bursitis, and a frozen shoulder capsule. She had ten treatments total with PSI. After the eighth one, I prescribed physical therapy. With the help of a very competent and knowledgeable physical therapist, Candice was able to get close to 100 percent range of motion back in that shoulder and she was finally pain free.

PSI AND HEADACHES

PSI pioneer Dr. Lyftogt says he has had remarkable success treating headaches with PSI in a very similar fashion to the one I used to treat Candice's frozen shoulder.[7] I have had a handful of headache cases that have responded well to this type of treatment, but I've also had a handful of cases where it's done nothing and others in which patients experienced mixed results. Before PSI, I treated headaches caused by muscle, tendon, or ligament problems with classic prolotherapy, hydrodissection of the greater occipital nerves deep in the neck muscles, manipulation, or some combination of these treatments.

Kim, one of my chronic headache patients, experienced some positive effects to everything I've tried with her, but nothing so far has fixed her. Kim was involved in a bicycle riding accident when she was twelve. She landed on her head and shoulder, broke her collarbone, and hurt her cervical spine. She has suffered from migraine headaches and other neck problems ever since. She had shoulder surgery, which alleviated some of her pain but did not help the headaches. Turning her head the wrong way can trigger a migraine. Kim reported she had been to neurologists who just kept increasing the drugs she took. She had gone to a cranial sacral specialist, to various massage therapists, and to physical therapists. The physical therapy brought on more headaches. She was frequently getting adjustments from her chiropractor,

"In the years I've been seeing you, my quality of life has definitely improved. I have always felt there is hope after your treatments."

but she did not have enough stability in her neck to hold the adjustments. Her chiropractor suggested she see me.

I did classic prolotherapy on her neck every five or six weeks for a year. Following this, she reported that the headaches had somewhat subsided. She continued to come back every six months for a tune up, and while that gave her some stability to her neck, she still suffered from migraine headaches. I recently did a new kind of platelet-rich plasma (PRP) treatment to the deep nerves in her neck called the greater occipital nerves. This has made the migraines abate, although Kim still gets occasional, more "garden variety" tension headaches. If she gets a headache that won't go away, she will come in and I will give her a deep nerve hydrodissection with low-dose dextrose and lidocaine, which will usually get rid of the headache within a few days. As of writing, I have just begun adding PSI to Kim's treatments, and she has experienced a very positive response.

Kim told me, "In the years I've been seeing you, my quality of life has definitely improved. I have always felt there is hope after your treatments. My neck pain, back pain, and headaches are all better. You were the first doctor who listened to me, looked at the anatomy of my neck, and found what my problems were. I would absolutely recommend the range of regenerative injection treatments to anyone in my position who is wandering around, wondering what is wrong."

PSI AND POST-CONCUSSION SYNDROME

Unfortunately, many athletes, often young ones, experience sports concussions. If it is a low-energy, acute concussion, 99 percent of patients will recover from it with good, old watchful waiting and brain rest. The real problem begins at a difficult-to-pinpoint time when an acute concussion instead becomes a full-blown post-concussion syndrome (PCS). PCS causes neurologic pain and headaches, often exacerbated by emotional issues, stem-ming both from the injury and from other sources.

Emily came to my practice with post-concussion syndrome that had been bothering her since her junior year in high school, when she suffered a severe concussion playing for her school's soccer team. Despite being aware of the dangers of a concussion, she was not forced to stop playing in the same game after she was knocked down hard by a much larger player. This trauma caused the concussion after her head bounced off the turf. The injury was severe enough that Emily had to miss about a month of school. That caused her additional stress because she was competing for an athletic scholarship.

When she returned to school, she kept up with a wide variety of extracurricular activities, despite the constant headaches she still suffered from the concussion. She tried treatments from both neurologists and integrative medicine practitioners to help her get over the headaches and the constant pain and anxiety they caused. Nothing helped.

A friend referred her to me because she had heard I had successfully dealt with this syndrome before. However, I was often frustrated because many of these young athletes would return to their previous athletic activities and suffer additional concussions. The problem is the more concussions either a child or an adult experiences, the more concussion-prone they become. It also takes them longer to recover from even minor concussions. After two or three serious concussions, the athlete is at much higher risk for PCS, and the other chronic neurologic problems that stem from this diagnosis.

Because of the degree of pain and tenderness Emily experienced, I referred her to a colleague who is an expert in PSI. In this situation, the first treatment is critical. If the patient does not experience at least a temporary lessening of symptoms, it is unlikely this treatment will help. Luckily, Emily did briefly feel better after her first treatment. As she progressed through the protocol, she began to experience longer periods of pain relief. It took longer than the expected eight treatments, but Emily eventually got to the point where she was free of pain most of the time. And, happily, she agreed she would no longer play soccer or other sports that would obviously put her in jeopardy for another concussion.

BIOPUNCTURE

Biopuncture uses biologically active substances to help regulate pain, swelling, inflammation, and toxic accumulation in the body. Unlike steroid injections or non-steroidal anti-inflammatory medications, which have many undesirable side effects, biopuncture is thought to help support natural healing mechanisms.[8] Biopuncture was first introduced in the early 1990s in Europe by Jan Kersschot, M.D., a Belgian family practice physician who was also trained in prolotherapy, acupuncture, neural therapy, homeopathy, and traditional approaches to musculoskeletal pain. While perineural superficial injections use low-dose dextrose or dextrose with lidocaine, biopuncture uses ultra-low-dose biologic, but not homeopathic, amounts of natural products like Traumeel, Lymphomyosot, or Zeel. These remedies are chosen for their anti-inflammatory, pain-relieving, and tissue-healing effects. They were formulated at the beginning of the twentieth century and have been safely used in Europe for almost one hundred years. In the last twenty years, instead of small pills or topical creams and gels, the formulas became available in liquid form. Dr. Kersschot combined his knowledge of conventional and complementary medicine, and began injecting the formulas with great success to treat common pain conditions such as tendonitis and arthritis.

Traumeel, which is one of the most common formulas utilized both orally and via injection, contains fourteen different ingredients including arnica, chamomile, calendula, belladonna, echinacea, and a few minerals.[9] Biopuncturists usually inject a mixture of natural products combined with a local anesthetic medicine like lidocaine. Products used in biopuncture, unlike those used in homeopathy, are not diluted to the extent that they contain no active product. These "micro-doses" produce clinical effects because they appear to stimulate the immune system and restart the healing capacity. Traumeel has been shown in studies to increase tissue-healing growth factors.[10]

Most commonly, injections are performed with a small needle just under the skin into the subcutaneous tissue (like PSI) or muscle. Biopuncture specialists will also inject into ligaments, tendons, or bone. The goal of biopuncture is to regulate and restore the body's healing processes in order to get a complete and natural healing of injured tissues. Symptomatic relief may take longer, especially for chronic cases. In acute injuries, such as sports injuries, Dr. Kersschot's research reports a "turbo effect" with positive effects apparent a few days after the first treatment. At the time of this writing, biopuncture is better known in Australia, New Zealand, Europe, and the West Coast of the United States. The majority of patients choose biopuncture because they are in pain which has not responded to treatment with conventional medications, or they prefer to treat their conditions with complementary and alternative medicine approaches. It seems to be a good adjunct to other methods of RIT.

There is another treatment method, which started in France and is now popular across Europe. It is called mesotherapy, and is similar to biopuncture. It is shallow injections, given intradermally (into the skin layer), rather than below the skin as in biopuncture. Perineural superficial injections, biopuncture, and mesotherapy are all related treatments, which definitely have an important place in the new healing paradigm.

CHAPTER NINE
UNDERSTANDING PLATELET-RICH PLASMA TREATMENT

If you have read or heard anything about RIT before, it most likely has been about platelet-rich plasma (PRP). In PRP, the patient's own blood is spun at high speed in a centrifuge to separate and concentrate the platelets, and then they are injected into the injured area. The platelets in this form of RIT initiate the same healing cascade that prolotherapy precipitates, but theoretically with a much stronger effect. PRP is the form of RIT most widely used at the time of this writing by top athletes. It is also the form of RIT treatment being researched in a number of universities and medical centers in various parts of the world.

PRP works at least as well as prolotherapy for most injuries and seems to work more quickly to get to the healing end point. Some patients experience as much healing with one PRP treatment as they would with two to three prolotherapy treatment sessions. The desired end result of a PRP treatment is the same as for any other RIT treatment: the anatomic and functional repair of an injured tendon, ligament, or joint allowing it to bear greater mechanical stress during activity without pain. These methods provide a viable treatment option for problems that don't have a very good natural healing response or good surgical outcome history.

PRP is more expensive than prolotherapy because it takes

longer to perform and involves a PRP kit that must be purchased by the treating physician. But it's not as expensive or invasive as adult stem cell injection (ASCI) treatments or surgery. So particularly for athletes who want to get back to play as soon as possible, it has become the current method of choice, often producing seemingly miraculous results.

The desired end result of a PRP treatment is the same as for any other RIT treatment: the anatomic and functional repair of an injured tendon, ligament, or joint allowing it to bear greater mechanical stress during activity without pain.

That was the case with Dennis, a semi-professional tennis player who injured his knee in such a way he had a piece of cartilage missing from the chondral joint surface of his medial femoral condyle. For about two years, whenever he played tennis, by the end of the game he would be hobbling, his knee would start swelling, and he would be limping at work the next day. He was reluctant to have surgery, so he asked his orthopedic surgeon if there was anything else he could do. His surgeon sent him to see me, and I treated him with PRP. After two treatments, Dennis had no pain or swelling, and less than a month after the second treatment he could play tennis without any problem. Three months after his last treatment, I ordered another MRI. The radiologist report showed that, compared with the original MRI, "Post-op changes show signs of healing." When I called the radiologist and told him the patient had not had surgery, but rather PRP, the doctor told me he had never seen cartilage grow like Dennis's had. He found it difficult to believe Dennis had not had surgery, the healing was so remarkable.

HISTORY OF PRP

PRP has been used since the 1950s to help heal bone grafts, as well as in other operations where it was easy to obtain the necessary amount of a patient's blood because the person was already anesthetized.[1] PRP injection work used to require the processing of about 500 milliliters of blood to get sufficient platelet-rich plasma to inject into an injury. Over time, better centrifuge machine kit systems and protocols have been developed which now require only about 20 to 60 milliliters of blood. This is a bit more than is normally drawn for a blood test, but a lot less than is re-

Post-op heart patients using PRP require fewer blood transfusions and less pain medication. They also heal more quickly and suffer significantly fewer infections.

quired when one donates a pint of blood for the Red Cross.

Modern centrifuge-centered PRP was initially used in the 1980s in the dental community to enhance wound healing in cancer patients who needed jaw reconstruction. The first report about PRP was published in 1987 and focused on a study of open-heart surgery patients for whom PRP was used to avoid excessive blood loss.[2] Until that time, platelets were considered to function primarily as an aid to clotting. However, this study indicated that the post-op heart patients using PRP required fewer blood transfusions and less pain medication. They also healed more quickly and suffered significantly fewer infections.

There were other early studies on the successful use of PRP treatment for chronic non-healing skin ulcers.[3] The patients in these studies had received standard wound care for an average of approximately four years. With the addition of platelet-derived growth factors, the mean time to 100 percent healing was decreased to a remarkable ten weeks. No abnormal cell growth or scar tissue was observed. Other researchers demonstrated that PRP greatly improved the success of skin grafts in burn patients.

Following these initial studies, the use of PRP exploded across many medical specialties. PRP has been used in cardiovascular surgery; neurosurgery; ophthalmology; urology; ear, nose, and throat surgery; and cosmetic surgery. It is now being used in sports medicine and orthopedic surgery. It is also being investigated for dry eyes, neurology, intervertebral disc problems, plastic surgery, bone regeneration, and gastric ulcers.

Treatment of musculoskeletal injuries with platelet-rich plasma in sports medicine was reported in a clinical research study by Allan Mishra, M.D., of Stanford University, who has successfully used this method to treat patients with chronic severe elbow tendinosis ("tennis elbow").[4] Patients had failed all conservative treatments including rest, NSAIDs, elbow straps, and steroid injections and were otherwise facing surgery. PRP injection was compared against local anesthetic injection. Only

10 percent of control subjects reported improvement. Patients receiving PRP were 60 percent better at eight weeks, 81 percent better at six months and 93 percent better at two years.[5] Although this was a weakly controlled pilot study, he was able to get it published in an elite sports medicine journal[6] and presented at worldwide conferences. He is currently running a much bigger trial that will hopefully add to the positive evidence that PRP works for tennis elbow.

Christopher Centeno, M.D., and John Schultz, M.D., established the Regenexx Clinic and system, which is the foremost stem cell-based musculoskeletal practice in the U.S., and also works with developing and researching PRP treatments.[7]

Other physicians interested in PRP include Neal ElAttrache, M.D., the Los Angeles Dodgers team physician and former physician for the Los Angeles Rams; Gerjo van Osch, Ph.D., an orthopedic researcher at Erasmus University Medical Center in the Netherlands; Samir Mehta, M.D., Chief of the Division of Orthopaedic Trauma at the Hospital of the University of Pennsylvania; Peter DeLuca, M.D., the Philadelphia Eagles team physician; and Michael Scarpone, D.O., from Alleghany Hospital in Pittsburgh, Pennsylvania, who serves as the team physician for the Pittsburgh Pirates.[8]

Although many of these physicians have only used PRP experimentally on one type of injury or another, they are all cautiously optimistic about the effect it can have on a variety of injuries.

THE FUNCTION OF PLATELETS

PRP is made from concentrated platelets derived from the patient's own blood. Platelets are one of the main types of cells in human blood, the other two being white and red blood cells.

When someone is injured, it is the function of the platelets to form a clot to stop bleeding and to release certain growth factors which activate the body's natural healing mechanisms. Inside platelets are alpha granules, which contain growth factors and bioactive proteins essential both for tissue repair and for healing. Platelets also contain chemicals that regenerate ligament and tendon fibers. All of these chemical messengers appear to exert a bio-regulatory action, which affects soft tissue repair, cartilage repair, inflammation, bone healing, wound healing, and post-operative blood loss. PRP has also been shown to have antibacterial and antifungal properties.

Allan Mishra, M.D., and other researchers at Stanford University in Palo Alto, California, have offered a commonly accepted medical hypothesis for PRP's mechanism of action on tendon, muscle and ligament healing.[9] They hypothesize PRP is delivered to the tissue in its inactivated form. The collagen in connective tissue activates the platelets, which then causes them to release the bioactive proteins and growth factors from their alpha granule. These chemical messengers signal genes to augment the healing stage and activate local stem cells. This causes stem cells to migrate from the local blood and bone marrow to the treatment site. The stem cells then trigger our body to create new cartilage, ligament, tendon, or muscle cells as needed at the injury site. At the same time, the cytokines and growth factors downgrade the local inflammation. They mitigate the internal war between the bad proteins, which slowly chew up the joint cartilage, eventually causing severe osteoarthritis, and the good proteins, which stop this degeneration. Without this help, in a typical knee with osteoarthritis it takes approximately five to ten years from symptom onset to knee replacement, which becomes necessary when the cartilage is gone and the knee joint is bone on bone.

Rinalda was close to that point. She saw me for a variety of problems for over a dozen years. When I did my first exam, focused on another area, I noticed she walked in a way that indicated knee problems. I had her get x-rays of her knees along with the other studies I ordered. She had mild arthritis in her left knee and moderate in her right.

After we resolved her tennis elbow with prolotherapy, she asked me to try it on her knees, which by then were interfering with her tennis game. Six treatments gave her substantial mobility and pain relief. She was even able to return to tennis. I continued to give her tune-ups, and, when the right knee was beginning to approach severe arthritis, I administered a series of PRP treatments. She agreed to take it easy until the healing process was finished, and she showed remarkable improvement. So she tried a few rounds of tennis. While playing one day, she turned quickly and noticed an immediate pain in her left knee, the one that prolo had helped up until that point. She stopped her game and came in to see me. Her knee was swollen, warm, and sore. Before trying any RIT, I sent her for an MRI, which showed a very severe tear of her meniscus. I agreed to try a PRP treatment and see what it could accomplish. Unfortunately, after two treatments, I saw no improvement. Her meniscus was really torn up.

Because this was prior to my using stem cell injections in my practice, I had to send her to a surgeon who removed her torn meniscus using arthroscopic surgery. Remember when I said that putting a scope in an arthritic joint was like sticking your hand in a hornet's nest? Well, Rinalda experienced that phenomenon. Her formerly better knee became her bad knee, forcing her to lead with her formerly bad knee going up and down stairs. We tried a steroid injection, viscosupplement injection, prolotherapy, and eventually we tried PRP. She did multiple rounds of physical therapy, both in the water and on land. When it finally calmed down and she was out of severe pain, tennis was out of the question and stairs were still a problem. Rinalda is currently weighing her financial ability to have ASCI against the potential problems of knee replacement. Nonetheless, she told me, "Hey, you have kept my knees working twice as long as other docs told me I could have expected. If I can hang in there, maybe I'll win the lottery, get ASCI, conquer stairs, and even get back to tennis."

THE PRP PROCEDURE

PRP is particularly effective when it is injected into the ends of tendons that naturally lose their blood supply as we age. Without sufficient blood flow, it is more difficult for healing to occur. By delivering the platelets exactly where they are needed, a PRP treatment promotes both soft tissue and bone healing in areas like those around the rotator cuff and the Achilles tendon. These are areas where the blood supply decreases as we age, hampering our ability to naturally repair them. When injured, these tendons can easily degenerate, tear and sometimes cause chronic pain.

The usual types of PRP procedures can be done in a doctor's office in thirty to sixty minutes, depending upon the type and severity of injury. Some athletes have reported being back to their game as quickly as two days after treatment, although three to ten days of downtime and six weeks away from rigorous training is the most common response to treatment.

PRP can be used in any situation where I could use prolotherapy. PRP treatment generally costs about twice as much as prolotherapy because of the extra equipment and time needed to prepare and administer the PRP solution. Most physicians who offer their patients both treatments reserve PRP for larger tendon and muscle tears, for severe ligament sprains, for any cartilage tear or defect, and for more advanced arthritis of a joint. Also critical to treatment selection is the size of the area being treated. Most large spine treatments require multiple injections into several ligaments. The standard amount of solution needed to perform a spine treatment could be anywhere between 10 and 40 milliliters, whereas the standard PRP solution obtained at one time is 7–10 milliliters. Consequently, if PRP is going to be used in a large area, its use will be reserved for the most injured segments. The rest of the area can be treated with prolotherapy during the same treatment session.

Ursula flew in from Austria to see me. She had been taking a large dose of hydrocortisone for severe adrenal failure and felt like her tendons and ligaments were falling apart. She reported being in chronic pain in many parts of her body. We went over her labs and her medical history. I performed a physical exam. She said, "I want you to treat me with the strongest thing you have." I said, "Well, the strongest thing I would use for your condition is PRP. I can do a large blood draw, and we can make almost as much PRP as we need to treat you." I made 30 milliliters of PRP out of 110 milliliters of whole blood for her, and treated her from the middle of her back up to the top of her neck. I also treated her wrist. I used prolotherapy solution to treat some of the areas for which I did not have enough PRP. Because she had flown over from Europe and could not return for follow up as easily as a more local patient, I did a more extensive treatment than usual. She had been all over the world looking for a solution for her chronic problems. When I finished treating her, I said, "That's enough. I've had it, you've had it, and we should stop." Following the treatment, she contacted me and reported her pain had begun to subside. She was making plans for a return trip.

PRP SOLUTIONS

Opinions vary about the optimal concentration of PRP. A body's normal platelet concentration is approximately 200,000 platelets per microliter of blood. Researchers recommend a minimum four- to five-fold increase in platelet concentration for an enhanced healing effect to occur.[10]

Not all PRP is the same. Effectiveness varies, depending on who's doing it, the systems they're using, and whether or not what they're doing actually constitutes a PRP treatment. Some doctors are injecting platelets, but PRP is concentrated platelets, at a minimum of four to five times the baseline concentration. Many doctors are not doing that.[11]

You can make PRP in a variety of different ways. There are a lot of variables the physician needs to understand in order for the treatment to be as effective as possible. Because of the system I am using now, and the extent of my education about the procedure, I can formulate PRP to correctly address each patient's problem. I can fine tune the concentration and have an accurate platelet count reading with the help of sophisticated laboratory cell-counting machines, so that I know exactly how concentrated the PRP injection is going to be. Many doctors have no clue either about this technology or about the extent of the science behind how PRP works. They have a one-size-fits-all model, using the same concentration of PRP for every patient who walks in the door, whatever their problem may be. When the physician doesn't customize the treatment to the individual patient, it's not surprising that PRP does not work as effectively as it could.

To place a PRP injection correctly, I have found ultrasound guidance valuable. However, at a meeting of sports medicine specialists that I recently attended in 2012, out of fifty doctors present, as few as eight of them were using ultrasound to guide their injections. Even fewer orthopedic surgeons use ultrasound. There has been a study showing that without such guidance, even a trained orthopedic surgeon only successfully places an injection into the knee joint 75–90 percent of the time.[12]

At the time of writing, there are over forty physicians in Philadelphia, many of them surgeons, who use PRP to some extent

---

The pioneers of regenerative healing are constantly working to develop better ways of performing PRP injections that are more effective for patients and cause less discomfort.

---

in their practice. I wonder whether some of these surgeons have noticed that medically aware patients have begun requesting PRP instead of surgery. Consequently, they are offering it.

I had a discussion with an orthopedic surgeon at a scientific dinner meeting, who told me, "Shiple, this stuff doesn't work. I just do it to appease them until they make up their mind that they're going to get surgery." It appears some doctors price PRP treatments as a "loss leader," charging less than they would for doing cortisone shots, just to keep patients in the practice.

The pioneers of regenerative healing are constantly working

to develop better ways of performing PRP injections that are more effective for patients and cause less discomfort following the procedure. Classic PRP produced by commercial centrifuge machines contains some red blood cells, along with the white blood cells and concentrated platelets. This is now known as "blood-filled" or "bloody" PRP. These red cells have been known to stimulate a strong inflammatory reaction in a patient's treated tissue. With some patients, this can necessitate potent pain medication and several weeks to recover from a treatment because of the excessive inflammation. There is anecdotal evidence that eliminating the red blood cells and white blood cells eliminates the excessive inflammation and severely painful treated tissue.[13] Patients recover from the treatment much more easily. This new preparation is known as "bloodless PRP." Many patients have told me that the switch from blood-filled to bloodless PRP made a big, positive difference in their recovery. However, some centrifuges and kits for concentrating platelets to produce bloodless treatments do not effectively concentrate platelets enough to fit the scientific definition of PRP. Unfortunately, ineffective, insufficiently concentrated PRP made from these kits has made its way into the orthopedic research arena, creating the appearance that PRP doesn't work.

HEALING TAKES TIME

Just as a single prolotherapy treatment initiates a long and gradual healing process, so does a PRP treatment. This does not mean a patient needs to take a lot of downtime to recuperate; rather, he needs to cut back on excessive activity while the injured tissue heals. I usually like patients to allow one or two days of rest, followed by at least a couple weeks of very curtailed exercise. This is all about healing properly, which takes time. There is always a fine line for a serious athlete between wanting to heal well and wanting to get back to his or her sport.

Jacob is a good example of respecting that line. An extremely successful businessman, Jacob was influential in founding and running one of the largest financial firms in the world. He was used to working more than ninety hours a week during his exec-

> "After five treatments, I was back to 100 percent. I cannot imagine a better outcome. I was able to compete in the Kona, Hawaii, Ironman in 2012."

utive years. He also played tennis and basketball. When he sold his company early in the 2000s, he was in his forties and full of energy, so he decided to become a runner. After four months of running, he participated in a short triathlon that occurred during a hurricane. Despite the darkness, rain, thunder, and lightning, he decided to finish the race. At that point, he realized he more than enjoyed it—he was hooked. Since then, he has completed over forty other triathlons, three Ironman races, and seven half-Ironman races. He trains twenty-five to thirty hours a week, every week of the year.

As most endurance athletes do, Jacob incurred injuries, mainly of his ankle and knee. He had been treated by one of the top doctors specializing in running in the country. He received cortisone shots, which did not help his condition. He had taken anti-inflammatory medication. He had been to a chiropractor, who had helped him, but had not been able to strengthen Jacob's injured joints enough to get him fully back into the sport. He had done physical therapy for two years and tried acupuncture. He felt he was out of options. It got to the point where the tendons and ligaments in his left ankle were so weak and stretched that he could barely stand up at his kitchen counter. As a result, the patella in his right knee became inflamed. Jacob was planning to compete in two Ironman races that year and hopefully qualify for the world championship Ironman in Hawaii. The long-term problem for Jacob was that every time he would get close to qualifying for Hawaii, one of his chronic injuries would get aggravated and prevent him from reaching his potential.

He went to one of the foremost orthopedic surgeons in the Philadelphia area. This physician told him that while reconstructive surgery could fix his knee and ankle, the surgery would make it impossible for him to continue competing in triathlons. He suggested Jacob see me. We discussed PRP and formulated a treatment plan that would allow Jacob to participate in both Ironman competitions.

I treated both his left ankle and right knee at the same time. He had five PRP treatments. "After the first treatment," Jacob told me, "I had significant improvement immediately. PRP allowed me to not miss a beat in my training, which is critical for triathlons, which require continuity. After five treatments, I was back to 100 percent. I cannot imagine a better outcome. I was able to compete in the two qualifying triathlons, which allowed me to participate in the Kona, Hawaii Ironman in 2012. It was a huge privilege to be there, and I owe my ability to do so to you, and to these treatments."

PRP FOR A SPORTS HERNIA

All athletes need core strength, but it is particularly essential for those playing professional soccer. Ryan, a two time MVP on the Baltimore Blast indoor soccer team, had always been a specimen of physical fitness. One day while playing he began to experience pain in his left side in his lower abdominal muscles and in the groin area. Over time, the pain began to spread to the right side. He went to the team physician and rated his everyday discomfort as being at level one or two on the ten-point pain scale, with zero being no pain and ten being the worst possible pain. However, he told the doctor that when he started running or kicking the ball, his pain would rise to level nine. The doctor diagnosed him as having a sports hernia and suggested surgery. His athletic trainer recommended he see me to discuss platelet-rich plasma injections (PRP). When I examined him and explained PRP, Ryan decided to give it a try.

In my first examination, I saw evidence of multiple areas of damage. There are three tendon areas that I treat for sports hernias. He had all three involved. I was looking for one problem and finding three or four problems in each tendon. I could see all of it with diagnostic ultrasound, and I could guide the needle into these specific damaged areas with precision.

Treating Ryan was very complex work that had to be done correctly. If I had missed some of these problem areas, he wouldn't have recovered as well as he did. PRP with ultrasound guidance is meticulous work; it's almost like microsurgery. I study the tissues, comparing the patient's pathology to what is normal, take my time to find each problem area, then accurately place the needle and inject the PRP. Then I move to the next spot. By treating the area this way, the body is induced to heal the entire area and not just part of it. Depending on the injury, the process can take up to an hour and a half to find all the problems, map out the treatment, and carry out my treatment plan.

Ryan had three PRP treatments. After the first, Ryan recounted, "Right away I noticed a positive result. The first couple of days I had discomfort. However, after the first week I started feeling not great but much better."

Ryan's first and second treatments were spaced six weeks apart. After his second PRP session, he noticed a very big difference and began performing much better in games. After each treatment, on my advice, Ryan rested for two days and then resumed his regular activities. He took one dose of the prescribed narcotic pain medication the day of the treatment and then did not need further pain medication, even though he was doing hard, vigorous exercises, jumping and kicking soon after treatment. Ryan really guided his own rehabilitation, and to be honest, pushed himself a lot harder than I would have recommended. Most of my elite athletes do that. They know their bodies well and usually bounce back rapidly from these treatments. As a recreational rather than elite athlete, when I had PRP it took eight weeks before I regained full range of motion and the ability to do light workouts. However my professional athlete patients frequently are back doing full workouts in just a couple of weeks. Ryan went through his next soccer season without experiencing any problems.

"After three treatments I felt 100 percent cured," Ryan told me, "I would tell athletes or anyone else that before they consider surgery I would definitely go with PRP. It is much safer and the healing process is shorter. For me, it was a very positive experience."

PRP FOR ROTATOR CUFF TEARS

Danielle, a woman in her forties, came to me with her right shoulder hurting badly. She reported that there was no trauma. She just woke up one morning and noticed pain in her shoulder. Within a few weeks, she had similar pain in the left shoulder. In her history, she told me she had had a lot of congenital problems with her spine and neck. She saw a chiropractor, who had kept her going for many years. He was not able to help her shoulder problem, so he sent her to me. Upon MRI and ultrasound examination, it appeared she had micro-tears that had built up over the years until they developed into a large, full-thickness rotator cuff tear in the right shoulder and a smaller, but significant one in the left.

Having worked most of her life as a paralegal for a personal injury lawyer, she had done a lot of computer work. Because of her shoulders, she was on temporary disability and could no longer go to the gym, where she enjoyed both spinning classes and weight training. Now she could not lift a pot off of the stove. Danielle felt she was running out of options. Because of her work in the personal injury field, she was reluctant to go to an orthopedic surgeon. "I do not like auto mechanic doctors who often misdiagnose and don't listen to you. I have recently talked to five people who had rotator cuff surgery. Two thought it was awesome. Three had real problems. That did frighten me. I was close to going on permanent disability. I don't think I'll ever be able to go back to weight training."

With the severity of her tears, I recommended going directly to PRP and also added a fat graft to fill the rotator cuff defect. The addition of a graft allows the growth factors to stay in the tissue defect while the tissue begins to repair. Danielle has had four PRP treatments, two sessions on the right shoulder and two on the left. I treated the tendon in her right shoulder and she report-ed it felt absolutely healed. I am still treating the left shoulder, which was less severely damaged than the right.

"Once the lidocaine is in, I just experience a feeling of pres-sure. I don't watch. I just focus on my breathing," Danielle told me. "I know I am going to have a couple of tough days, but I have learned how to prepare for them. After those painful days, I have been getting steady improvement with PRP. I have been recom-mending you to lots of people. You are a straight shooter and do not make me feel stupid. I am extremely happy with the decision I made. The right shoulder had been my bad shoulder. Now it is the good one. I have full range of motion and can lift with it. It is real improvement. I am not just masking pain. It is slow, steady improvement. I haven't achieved full recovery yet with my left shoulder, but I am hopeful. I would recommend it to anybody, and would tell them to try prolotherapy or PRP before opting for surgery. The therapeutic idea makes sense to me: work with your body's own natural healing abilities."

CHAPTER TEN
UNDERSTANDING ADULT AUTOLOGOUS STEM CELL INJECTION (ASCI) TREATMENTS

S tem cells are the exciting vanguard of a new frontier in medicine, one which holds great promise for helping or curing injuries and diseases that were previously considered incurable. Adult autologous stem cell injection (ASCI) treatment has vast potential in many medical fields, including musculoskeletal medicine.

While stem cell treatments have been used successfully in many parts of the world for several decades,[1] they have not been very widely used in the United States for a variety of reasons. One is the ongoing debate about embryonic stem cells, also called autogenic stem cells. Many people do not realize that getting autogenic stem cells, unless there is a perfect donor match, may require lifelong use of anti-rejection drugs, which are both expensive and potentially toxic.

Autogenic stem cells are irrelevant to the work I do because I only work with autologous stem cells, cells that come from the body of the patient I'm treating. There are many types of stem cells in our bodies. The kinds I most often use to treat patients are a combination of hematopoietic stem cells (HSCs), mesenchymal stem cells (MSCs), blastomeric stem cells, and very small embryonic-like stem cells (VSELs).

The two most common sources of stem cells used to treat patients with musculoskeletal conditions are bone marrow and adipose tissue, or fat, usually taken from a patient's buttock or abdomen area. For the same-day procedures new treatment-paradigm practitioners are now performing, we try to maximize the amount of MSCs we get from a given patient, because it now appears, ac-

The stem cell is the director of the healing process.

cording to new research, they are the most important stem cells for healing cartilage, bone, ligament, and tendon.[2] When I harvest stem cells from bone marrow, I normally get millions to hundreds of millions of all types of stem cells per milliliter of bone marrow. Of these, the smallest percentage is MSCs. There are about 500 to 1,000 times more stem cells in fat than in bone marrow, and many more of them are MSCs. How many more depends, in part, on the age and body composition of a given patient. Some athletes have such a low percentage of body fat that I have to tell them to eat a little more in the weeks before the procedure.

There are two methods of utilizing fat in a regenerative treatment. One is to use raw fat that has been extracted using a mini-liposuction procedure. This becomes the scaffold structure that the stem cells can cling to while waiting to adhere to the target area of tissue I am trying to help heal. The other, called the stromal vascular fraction (SVF) method, is to extract the stem cells from the raw fat by digesting the fat away through a chemical or mechanical process, leaving behind the pure stem cells. However, as of December 2011, the FDA has made it illegal for doctors in the United States to make fat-derived stem cells without getting a new drug license.[3] Without a major policy shift or being part of an FDA-approved research protocol, it is extremely unlikely that the FDA will clear fat-derived stem cell treatment as a viable legal option for use in clinical practice.

When I harvest stem cells, I may get hundreds of thousands of usable mesenchymal stem cells from a patient's stem cell sample. In countries where it is legal to grow them in a lab, the culture can yield tens of millions. This allows doctors in those countries to treat more severe disease and/or larger areas more effectively with a single treatment. To be fair, the FDA does have a duty to protect all of us from unsafe drugs and to make sure the distribution of drugs across state lines is done safely. However, those of us who practice cellular medicine in the United States do not feel the FDA should be involved in regulating how patients and doctors decide to use each patient's tissue in the treatment of that patient.

LIVING WITH ARTHRITIS

Cheryl was one of my first stem cell patients. I had already treated her severely arthritic right knee with three PRP treatments. She got enough relief to be able to successfully manage most activities of daily life for a month or two before needing to run back to the doctor's office to have her knee drained. But she wanted to see if she could improve enough to do some sort of exercise again to fight the weight gain that had come with diminished activity. She held up well with the procedure, which took over two hours. She told me she felt pressure when I "harvested" her bone marrow, but that it wasn't particularly painful. She left the office after the treatment using crutches because it was essential to keep weight off of her knee as much as possible for the first two days to allow the stem cells time to adhere to the treated area. Cheryl is not a fan of narcotic painkillers since they generally make her nauseous within the first couple of doses. I strongly recommended she take them after this treatment, and she did. She had enough pain to continue the narcotic medication for three days. She then switched to acetaminophen. She used the crutches for four days, and then only needed a cane. Most of her swelling had resolved by that time, and she was able to put in a fairly full workday.

"Comparing ASCI to the hip replacement I had over ten years ago," she told me, "this was far easier. Within a week, I was capable of driving and resumed many of my usual activities. Two weeks after the procedure, I felt capable of going to a pool and gently exercising my legs. A month after the procedure, my knee looked more normal than it had in years: less swollen and bumpy. I felt more stable when walking. My range of motion was good and there was no heat emanating from the joint." At the time of writing, three years have passed since her treatment, and Cheryl is still functioning well with her treated knee. She still has arthritis, but she is able to live with it.

HOW STEM CELLS WORK

A PRP solution, made from the patient's blood, contains some stem cells as well as growth factors and cytokines, proteins that affect inflammation and other cell communication. These signal the body to heal a tendon or ligament tear or to help heal small injuries in cartilage. PRP works by indicating to your body's own stem cells that they should come and help heal an injury. On the other hand, autologous stem cells have the ability to attach to the damaged tissue and turn it into healthy tissue, repairing the defect in question. The treatments are much more concentrated, making the process many times stronger than PRP.

The stem cell is the director of the healing process. When stem cells are injected into an injured area, either as part of a PRP or ASCI treatment, they adhere to the abnormal tissue and become whatever specifically is needed to help heal the injury. These stem cells can become fibroblasts, which form new collagen, or chondrocytes, which form new cartilage. They also attract additional platelets from the local blood supply, which, with the fibroblasts, start the process of growing new connective tissue, cartilage, or bone. The cells also activate bioactive proteins and growth factors, which signal more stem cells to come in. The more concentrated the stem cells are, the higher the potential for full healing.

I used to think that the number of MSCs determined the effectiveness of a treatment. Now I have seen evidence presented, both at conferences and in articles, that it may not be the absolute number of MSCs that determines whether or not patients can grow cartilage or heal other tissues which are difficult to repair.[4] As of the time of writing, the most current thinking is that the mesenchymal stem cells do not act alone. They need the platelets, they need the growth factors and cytokines from the platelets, and they need other types of stem cells. They also need the right environment for the cells to work, hence the PRP pre-treatment before stem cell treatment has been introduced. This new model hypothesizes that the MSC is the project manager and the hematopoietic stem cells (HSCs), found in much greater numbers, are the workers. Consequently, it's not one cell line responsible for healing the tissue, but rather a mixture of cells, each with their own part in this complicated ballet.

Besides the project managers (MSCs) and the workers (HSCs), there is another element necessary to complete the task—the scaffolding. Currently, doctors use either raw fat from the patient or bovine collagen as the scaffold material. Other scaffolding materials are in development by several companies at the time of writing.

HOW AN ASCI PROCEDURE IS DONE

In the most commonly used stem cell procedure, the first part of the process is to draw the blood needed for PRP, which is administered in combination with the stem cells. While the centrifuge procedure is in progress, the physician harvests stem cells, usually from the patient's pelvic bone, using ultrasound or x-ray to guide the needle. The physician most often uses a long-acting and strong numbing agent that numbs everything from the outer layer of skin to the membrane covering the bone. Patients usually report feeling pressure rather than discomfort or outright pain. This is not necessarily the case if the patient has a history of low back pain. Such patients may feel more pain than others because the superficial cluneal nerves that lie underneath the skin over the buttock may be hyper-irritated and more sensitive.

My associates at Regenexx, the clinic that has done the most research work developing this type of treatment, have found the amount of stem cells extracted can be significantly increased by only taking a small amount of bone marrow from each site where the harvesting needle pierces the wall of the bone marrow cavity.[5] The stem cells, particularly the MSCs, tend to adhere to the bone right where the needle pokes through the wall of the bone. The bone marrow needle is placed in more than one site to make sure the stem cells obtained for the procedure are as concentrated as possible. If the physician plans to use raw fat as a graft for the procedure, this is usually obtained after the bone marrow is drawn and placed in the centrifuge to separate the raw fat from any blood and oil obtained during the mini-liposuction technique.

> The beginning of the ASCI healing process takes about six weeks, but healing continues for six to twelve months or more.

The physician then applies a pressure dressing to the patient's buttock or abdomen to minimize bruising while the stem cells run through the same centrifuge used for PRP, although they are spun at a different rate. An automatic stem cell counter indicates the amount and type of stem cells per milliliter. The doctor injects the stem cell and PRP solutions into the site being treated using high-resolution diagnostic ultrasound or C-arm fluoroscopic x-ray guidance, which allows him to see the needle going precisely into the correct spot in the damaged area. In order for the cells to have a healing effect in the target tissue, they must be delivered accurately. From beginning to end, the procedure can take up to two hours and thirty minutes to treat one joint.

The pain following the procedure is significant enough to usually warrant several days' worth of prescription pain medication. Some of the pain is due to the extraction of the stem cells or fat, and in some patients, it may be due to the ASCI injections, especially if the injured tissue is a damaged tendon.

HEALING TAKES TIME

The beginning of the ASCI healing process takes about six weeks, but healing continues for six to twelve months or more. When injecting into a joint to stimulate cartilage growth, which is a particularly long-term process, we want to give the stem cells the chance to fully adhere to the injury site. We want the patient non-weight bearing for two days, and then partial-weight bearing for one to two weeks, until he can walk without a limp. To accomplish this, we use boots, unloading braces, or other appropriate devices to support the area. The patient is allowed to do gentle activities and range-of-motion exercises, but not vigorous exercises until about two to four weeks have passed.

There can be swelling for seven to ten days, and the patient can experience stiffness and pain during this period. Some discomfort can continue for a month or more. It takes three months before we can measure the clinical success of the procedure. The stem cells need that much time to begin to create as much new and healthy tissue as possible. Patients can see visible results as soon as a month after they are treated. After the pain has ceased, good rehabilitation is a critical next step.

This basic stem cell procedure is constantly being refined as I and other doctors involved with its development find ever more effective ways of using adult autologous stem cell injection treatments. I have been using this method since early 2010 on an ever-increasing basis for an expanding variety of injuries and musculoskeletal degenerative conditions. I anticipate seeing major advances in this field on a continuing basis. This treatment is so new there are no definitive studies, although a number are in progress, both in this country and in other parts of the globe.

My stories of patients who have undergone ASCI treatments

are also ongoing. At the time of writing this book, sufficient time has not yet elapsed to have definitive outcomes for procedures I have done on some of the patients whose stories I will share in this chapter. To keep up with both patient stories and advancements in the field of autologous stem cell injections, check my website at www.regen4life.com.

STEM CELLS FOR LESIONS, TEARS, AND FRACTURES

I treated Leonard, a martial arts expert who had injured his shoulder while competing, using his own stem cells. The force of the injury caused one bone to jab into another, leaving a full-thickness cartilage defect down to the bone surface. Leonard had first gone to his usual sports medicine doctor, who took him through the old treatment-paradigm methods. He was still experiencing significant pain, so that doctor suggested he see me. Since stem cells have the best chance of re-growing missing cartilage, I suggested them as the preferred treatment.

After the ASCI treatment and the initial recuperation period, all of Leonard's pain abated. He also showed signs of re-growing his cartilage on a nine-month follow-up MRI. The MRI reported an 80 percent filling in of the full-thickness hyaline cartilage defect. At the time of writing, he is approaching the twelve-month mark that would allow me to reevaluate the extent of his ability to resume his activities. Leonard was relieved at being pain free and able to pursue his passion in martial arts.

Denny is a runner in his early thirties. He came to me with a bad ankle injury. I performed three PRP treatments to treat a severe osteochondral lesion in the top of the talus bone in his ankle joint. The MRI showed a sizable defect where the surface cartilage was missing, and also showed a moderate amount of edema (swelling of the bone) under this lesion. After the treatments, he was completely asymptomatic, but had not yet tried to run. Using a repeat MRI, I did not see any cartilage growth from these treatments. I sent him to a specialist in New York City who was set up to do stem cell treatments inside the ankle joint through arthroscopic surgery. To do this, he would drill a hole into the ankle bone where the bone edema indicated the surrounding bone was dying and just below where the cartilage was missing, giving the stem cells an improved environment in which to grow.

This surgeon said Denny wasn't a candidate for that procedure, and instead suggested performing microfracture surgery, in which he would make several pin-holes over the damaged ankle bone with a sharp surgical tool and hammer. In this procedure, the ankle joint has to be pulled apart to give the surgeon access to the area where the cartilage is missing. The goal of this procedure is to stimulate the growth of scar cartilage called fibrocartilage. What we were born with is called hyaline cartilage. If it stays intact, hyaline cartilage can last our entire life without breaking down. Fibrocartilage lasts only three to five years before degenerating. At that point, the patient is back to bare bone, causing a rapid progression of osteoarthritis or degenerative arthritis. Either of these could lead to further disability, surgeries and chronic pain.

After this surgery, Denny would have developed symptoms of severe arthritis, probably before he was forty years old. Then his options would be limited to either fusion or joint replacement. Denny did not like this scenario, so he came back to me. At that point, we decided to try the stem cell treatment. Denny was at a similar point in his recovery to Leonard at the time of writing.

I treated Brent, a former Division I soccer player who continued to play in a semi-professional league after college, for a complete tear in his Achilles tendon. He sustained this injury during a match when another player accidentally kicked him in the back of his heel. He had already been treated with a surgical intervention called the "Topaz procedure." In this, the surgeon exposes the paratenon (the covering of the Achilles tendon). He then uses an infrared heat source device to burn away the abnormal nerves and blood vessels that are believed to cause or contribute to the tendon disease. This procedure seems to work with mild to moderate disease, but not with severe disease or a large tear, like Brent had. Brent felt a little better, went to physical therapy, and went back to soccer. His tendon quickly tore again, more severely than it had initially. He had several more treatments of different kinds, including PRP with a physician near his home. His tendon never healed. It was badly torn, and he was in chronic pain for a year and a half.

Brent found me through the Internet and came for my opinion. Given the treatments he had already failed, I suggested we go directly to ASCI. I treated him once, and after four weeks, he reported he was about 50 percent better. When I repeated his MRI six months later, his Achilles tendon looked like it was turning back into a normal tendon. He underwent one more stem cell treatment four months later, and upon radiological examination, his Achilles tendon was continuing to heal properly. He is now pain free and able to play soccer again without problems.

TREATING AVASCULAR NECROSIS

Randy had a condition that required prolonged steroid use. What can happen in this circumstance is that the patient develops what is called a "fatty liver," which means the liver doesn't process fat correctly, so some of it gets emptied into the blood-stream. These fat molecules can clog up the artery system in the hip, cutting off the blood supply. In effect, the hip bone dies where it meets the joint socket. This is called avascular necrosis (AVN) of the hip. Any bone that loses its blood supply can suffer bone death, or osteonecrosis.

Taking steroids on a long-term basis presents a significant risk factor for AVN or osteonecrosis. Performing multiple corti-sone injections on a patient increases the patient's risk of devel-oping AVN. An organization called the International Spine In-tervention Society (ISIS) has developed a guideline that dictates that no more than 210 milligrams or up to five injections' worth of triamcinolone, a common medium-potency injectable steroid, should be given to a patient per year to minimize the risk of de-veloping AVN or other complications.

That is exactly what had happened to Randy. He called to talk with me about treating the condition with stem cells. The proper procedure for this is to get the stem cells inside the head of the femur, a process in which I was about to be trained by an out-of-town colleague. Fortuitously, it turned out that Randy lived in the town where my colleague practiced. I arranged for him to be treated with the help of my colleague Michael Scarpone, D.O., one of the top experts in the country who performs this procedure.

The procedure went very smoothly. Randy was only twen-ty-six years old. We caught his AVN before the bone death was extensive enough to cause the head of the femur to collapse. Once the head begins to collapse, the success rate of any treatment we have to offer, including surgery, begins to decline significantly.

Following Randy's treatment, I received calls from numer-ous other people who needed this procedure. Without it, their only alternative would have been surgical decompression, where the surgeon puts a large drill bit into the femur head of the dying bone to try to re-establish blood supply to help the necrotic bone heal. This treatment is far less successful than treating with stem cells promises to be. Stem cells can cause the dying bone to regenerate back into normal bone with a normal blood supply. I predict that, as long as we diagnose a patient early enough in his disease process, bone marrow derived stem cells will help eradicate this condition for most of our patients.

Philippe Hernigou, M.D., is an orthopedic surgeon in France who has been performing AVN work since the 1990s with bone marrow-derived stem cells. Dr. Hernigou reports that even if the bone has collapsed, stem cell treatment can still help, but the percentage of good- to excellent outcomes falls off rapidly.[6]

STEM CELLS TO TREAT ARTHRITIS

Nina had run track in high school and college and had lost a lot of her cartilage from wear and tear or just overuse. She loved running so much that she kept doing so until she badly tore her meniscus while jogging when she was in her early thirties. The orthopedic surgeon she saw found advanced arthritis behind her kneecap and on the inside portion of her medial knee joint space. She underwent two arthroscopic surgeries, one to remove her damaged meniscal cartilage and another in which the surgeon performed microfracture on her femoral condyle. Both of these failed. She was left with chronic pain, and frequent swelling and locking of her knee. She did not want to get a joint replacement before forty, especially since she was caring for her three small children. Nina had been getting her knee drained every two weeks for two years when she came to me. I did four PRP treatments on her, following which she only needed her knee drained every two months. Still, her knee would swell if she jogged or just chased her kids around the house.

I suggested a stem cell treatment. After one, her knee never needed to be drained again. We did three treatments at three-month intervals. She also had a painful bone spur, which I removed in the course of her treatment with a large bone marrow-extraction needle and cannula with ultrasound guidance. That was her last remaining spot of pain, and it never came back. She has remained pain free and has had no further swelling since her first treatment more than three years ago. She began doing fitness walking and taking Zumba and Spinning classes, and working out with a trainer. She lost about thirty pounds and felt great. She told me, "My knees just don't hurt anymore. They feel normal." Although she had really good pain-management and range-of-motion outcomes, when I ordered another MRI twelve months after these first treatments, it showed no cartilage growth at all!

Nina's case is what led me to research Regenexx, the system I am now using for PRP and ASCI. The Regenexx Clinic and system has had more stem cell orthopedic experience than any other clinic in the United States. The doctors there are also leaders in presenting stem cell therapy for orthopedic injuries in terms of research, presentations, publications, and academic achievements.[7, 8, 9] Regenexx Sciences has pioneered musculoskeletal stem cell use at a very high clinical level. After researching their methods and results among several others, I determined they have the best system currently in use in the United States. Because I realized that Nina's lack of cartilage would eventually catch up with her, I asked her to consider a round of Regenexx treatments. She agreed, and her Regenexx ASCI treatment went very well.

I became the second Regenexx affiliate in early 2012. When doing ASCI, we use a group of treatments that consists of a pre-treatment with a type of PRP, or even prolotherapy, to calm the joint down to provide the stem cells with a much healthier joint environment. Within one week, we perform the stem cell treatment and follow that up within one to two more weeks with a PRP treatment. There are a variety of ASCI protocols being performed in the United States at the time of this publication. Some require administering the ASCI first, followed by either one or two PRP treatments within the next two months. Until we have head-to-head studies comparing each protocol, we won't be able to say absolutely which protocol is most effective.

Violet was my first Regenexx stem cell case. In my initial examination of her, I saw both a torn meniscus and bone-on-bone arthritis in her left knee. She didn't look like a good candidate for any form of RIT. She had pain going down her inner leg from her thigh to her ankle. When I looked at her films, the cause seemed to be continued use of a bone-on-bone arthritic knee, exacerbated by superficial pain of the saphenous nerve, which surrounds and travels very close to the main support ligament at the inside portion of the knee joint. Meniscal tears are common in patients with severe arthritis. Because the knee is bone on bone, it is easy for the meniscus to tear and herniate right out of the joint. Violet was also overweight, which put more pressure on her arthritic knee. Doctors had given her cortisone and viscosupplement injections, but these had not worked. She desperately wanted to avoid a joint replacement.

I agreed to try a PRP treatment, as well as a few PSI treatments, which took away her inner-leg saphenous nerve pain completely. She was left with bone-on-bone, joint line pain and pain from the herniated, torn meniscus on the inside of her knee. Based on the result of the initial PSI and a single PRP, I recommended I treat her with an ASCI treatment. I used a herniated meniscus protocol developed by a colleague of mine, David Crane, M.D. The protocol has since been modified by one of the Regenexx developers, Ronald Hanson, M.D. The protocol calls for a combination ASCI, PRP plus a fat graft injected between the medial collateral ligament (MCL) and the herniated meniscus. This graft acts as a bolster, or buttress, to push the herniated meniscus back into the joint. Part of the treatment was then directed at the MCL to make it strong and stable, and part of it was injected into the joint to treat the advanced arthritis.

Violet was placed in an unloader brace to open the joint on the inside of the knee. This brace gives the stem cells a chance to adhere and to survive the abnormal pressure put on the area of severe joint space narrowing. It also allows the herniated meniscus to stay inside the joint and heal. She had very little pain right after the procedure and only a bit more a few days following. A week or so after, her knee pain was gone. She had a brief return of pain a few months after, but it did not stem from the meniscus. The meniscus tear healed, and the meniscus was back in its correct position and no longer herniated. Using ultrasound to diagnose, I determined the pain was stemming from her still irritated saphenous nerve. When I treated her with PSI, the pain was entirely gone. After her first ASCI treatment, she wore the unloader brace for six weeks, and then only wore it as needed. She subsequently took trips to the Florida Keys and to Disney World, which required a lot of walking. Despite this, she continued to be pain free.

Six months after that first treatment, Violet was still pain free.

She had also followed a weight management program we recommended and has lost over fifty pounds. She was considering doing another stem cell cycle to encourage more cartilage to grow. Violet said these treatments had already changed her life. I told her that even though she was pain free for the time being the best thing for her knee was to continue treatment, if she could afford to do so. My best educated guess, given my experience and that of my Regenexx associates and other experts from around the world, is if I did one treatment of stem cells a year for five years, it might improve her chances to re-grow cartilage more so than if I did one treatment every three to five years. I believed the worst-case scenario would be that even if she did not re-grow cartilage she would maintain good pain control and function. That is still a good outcome for someone with severe arthritis.

HELPING ASCI WORK

To get the best result from ASCI, a patient needs to rest the injured area, keep weight off a weight-bearing joint for a few days, limit activity for a few weeks, and be aware of several other crucial dos and don'ts. Specific information about nutrition and medication is in Chapter Thirteen, and it is critical that patients considering ASCI consult that list at least one to three months before their stem cells are harvested. This will allow ample time to consult prescribing physicians about medications that could interfere with the treatment. It will also allow the opportunity to make the necessary additions to supplements and modifications to diet.

In this treatment, our knowledge of what will or won't affect the outcome of the procedure is evolving rapidly. Consequently, one can find a lot of information on the Internet, only some of which is helpful. For example, one patient read online that lidocaine had been shown to kill stem cells in culture. He came to me to discuss treatment and said, "If the lidocaine could be harmful to my stem cell treatment, don't give me any. I'll get through the procedure."

Other patients are very concerned about the level of pain they will experience with a stem cell procedure. I have found that if lidocaine is used at the surface of the skin and carried to the tissue layer near but not in the joint, the patient does not experience more than minimal discomfort with the procedure. Other patients have even eschewed short-term narcotic pain relief after reading that the more narcotic medication a patient gets, the more his testosterone goes down. There is research showing that good, healthy testosterone levels help control and direct healing processes in general and also help modulate our patients' pain perception.[10, 11]

I'm sure as we treat more patients we will learn more about who will respond well to the treatment, and what we can do to ensure this positive response. At the time of this writing, there remains a lot to learn in this regard. I have noticed thus far that some people who look like bad candidates for the treatment, such as Violet, sometimes do very well with it. Others who look like perfect candidates have not always done as well as I expected they would.

WHEN TO USE ASCI

My patient Gladys asked me to use stem cells to treat arthritis in her thumb. Two hand surgeons had already told her she needed surgery. She actually had moderate arthritis, not severe, but she was in a lot of pain. I convinced her to start with PRP. I told her that I think of the different forms of RIT as treating mild, moderate, and severe disease. I would advise prolotherapy as the proper treatment for mild disease, PRP for moderate disease, and stem cells for severe disease. I like to start with prolotherapy or PRP and ask the patient to consider moving up to a stronger treatment if they're not having a good clinical response. Stem cells are the strongest treatment I have in my toolbox to be able to offer someone who has advanced arthritis in a joint, to encourage the growth of cartilage in a joint, or to heal an extremely damaged tendon or ligament. Only occasionally are they the place to start.

I told Gladys she was a candidate for stem cells, but a better one for PRP. If it worked, she would get good relief for at least six to twelve months before I needed to do a tune-up treatment. Still, she wanted to know if the stem cells would cure her outright.

I said, "We're not curing arthritis yet with our stem cell treatment, but we are getting longer improvement with stem cells compared to anything else. A patient with moderate to severe arthritis is likely to experience anywhere from eighteen months to three to five years of relief from ASCI. PRP should give relief for nine to twelve months with one series of treatments. If we can give the patient three to five years of relief with ASCI, even though this procedure is more expensive than PRP, it still may prove more cost effective."

STEMS CELLS: THE ANATOMIC HOLY GRAIL?

The anatomic Holy Grail would be something that can cure what has been thought incurable—re-grow what was considered irreplaceable—and right now, stem cells certainly seem to be the foremost contender for the title. There is prolotherapy research going on in Argentina where surgeons, under the direction of researcher Gaston Topol, M.D., are looking in the joints of arthritic knees and hips using arthroscopic surgery, staining the joint cartilage and taking a biopsy of the diseased area.[12] Following this procedure, these patients are getting their arthritic joints injected with hypertonic dextrose prolotherapy solution six times throughout the year. At the end of the study, the surgeons are performing a second-look procedure with arthroscopic surgery. They are finding evidence of normal hyaline cartilage growth. Just simple dextrose is being injected, and it is creating cartilage buds, the beginning of new cartilage growth.

If dextrose is injected over years, will those cartilage buds coalesce and cover the entire joint with good cartilage? This research has shown that prolotherapy can encourage cartilage growth. Other research has shown that PRP can significantly concentrate growth factors.[13] So the potential for cartilage growth with PRP should be as good as or, hopefully, much better than with plain dextrose.

Think of the potential for stem cells, which have the power to self-renew. If you put a group of stem cells into a target area like an arthritic joint, and you can get those cells to stick to the damaged part of the joint, the stem cells will potentially keep replicating and multiplying on that damaged site. As they do so, they have the genetic ability to turn into the tissue that is needed for self-repair.

In the search for the "anatomic Holy Grail," the hope is if stem cells can grow cartilage and reverse arthritis, they could literally obviate the need for joint replacement surgery for millions of patients. We're not there yet, but in theory, in limited case reports, and in some case series projects, this goal seems to be a viable, possible outcome in the not-too-distant future.

In areas of the world where researchers can legally culture mesenchymal stem cells, scientists are growing a few thousand MSCs into tens of millions, which can then be injected into patients' joints. The higher the number of MSCs, the better the possibility to grow new tissue in difficult areas, such as inside a joint or between discs in the spine. Whoever can come up with the right cocktail to consistently get cartilage growth in an arthritic joint is going to have the best tool to treat these patients and will have found the real "Holy Grail" for arthritis.

In countries where it is legally permissible to utilize stem cell cultures, some amazing research is being done. For instance, the Regenexx group has opened a cultured stem cell lab in the Cayman Islands, where the Ministry of Health is supportive of their work. China, South Korea, Spain, Japan, Germany, Italy, Great Britain, Ireland, the Netherlands, Australia, New Zealand, the Caribbean, Mexico, Peru, Argentina, El Salvador, and other countries all have research projects with stem cells.

At stem cell conferences, new-paradigm practitioners give presentations on the newest advances in musculoskeletal research. Additionally, specialists in other fields lecture about how they have used stem cells to treat a variety of other ailments, from spinal cord and permanent nerve injuries to autism.

Researchers have had success working with patients with cerebral palsy, multiple sclerosis, and Parkinson's disease.[14, 15, 16, 17] One of the studies presented at the International Cellular Medicine Society (ICMS) annual research symposium in Las Vegas in 2010 showcased a group of interventional radiologists from Peru. They presented a case series study[18] with end-stage Parkinson's patients who could barely walk, talk, communicate, dress, or feed themselves. After one treatment of infusing the patients' concentrated bone marrow into their carotid artery (the main blood supply to the brain), they were able to show before and after treatment videos of these advanced end-stage Parkinson's patients with most of their symptoms lessened or reversed to the point of an apparent cure.

Other researchers have been treating people with autism using stem cells.[19] In August 2012, the FDA approved a small study in California in which thirty autistic children began treatment

---

In countries using stem cell treatments, doctors are treating conditions that cost us hundreds of billions of dollars to treat with other means in the United States.

---

with autologous stem cells harvested from their own banked umbilical cord blood.[20]

Stem cells are also proving useful in treating diabetes and the non-healing diabetic ulcers this disease can cause. There are stem cell clinics in Japan, Spain, and South America that are injecting a patient's own stem cells either into the blood vessels around the heart or into a peripheral vein to treat severe congestive or end-stage heart failure.[21] With just one to two treatments, doctors at the conference reported patients going from needing a heart transplant to undertaking a full exercise program with their own successfully treated heart.

In countries using stem cell treatments, doctors are treating conditions that cost us hundreds of billions of dollars to treat with other means in the United States. It is very possible we could get our healthcare costs under control if we simply opened up the doors to stem cell research and let our doctors start using the protocols used elsewhere in the world.

However, there is a dispute in the United States between the FDA and doctors trying to help their patients with their patients' own stem cells. The pharmaceutical industry also has a large stake in this issue, since companies are looking to develop these stem cell treatments into drugs that will become products, which could generate huge returns on research investments.

I am concerned that the question of profit will stand in the way of developing stem cell treatments. For example, the billions of dollars that are being spent to treat complications of diabetes—such as diabetic ulcers and vascular insufficiency, which leads to amputations, blindness, and kidney failure—are fueling a huge industry of resources and people. If we could cure diabetes by injecting a patient's own stem cells into the artery that supplies the pancreas, this may no longer be the case. This is being done in mainland China and in Brazil.[22]

While research in this field is still in its infancy and we have a distance to run until we cross the proverbial finish line, autologous stem cells have already demonstrated phenomenal early results in many areas of medicine. Imagine what wonders could lay ahead in this field. Unfortunately, these possibilities are mired in the courts of Washington, D.C. My hope is that we can raise funds from our successfully treated patients, our own clinics and the public to fund physician-designed and -run research studies that do not incur the millions to billions in futile research costs, which are currently the standard in the pharmaceutical industry. With such funding, the practice of medicine and the doctor-patient relationship could win out in the end. If it does, what you do with your cells will remain, as it should, a decision between you and your doctor.

CHAPTER ELEVEN
TREATING INJURIES WITH THE NEW PARADIGM

W hen I think about treating injuries with these new methods, I immediately picture some of the athletes I see. Athletes get injured with regularity and are aggressive in their treatment, usually coming to see me as soon as possible. When an injury is in the acute stage, I have available to me the full range of treatment and the ability to use each at the best possible time. An athlete knows his body well and is determined to get back to his regular workout routine as soon as possible. He is willing to push the envelope and wants the latest and fastest methods of healing. He comes to me and says he doesn't want to waste time on conservative care. Sometimes I need to slow him—or her—down.

That was necessary with Craig, a teenage basketball player who came to me with a moderately sprained ankle. He was accompanied by his father, whom I had previously treated with prolotherapy. Neither Craig nor his father wanted him to sit out any games, so they wanted me to immediately treat his ankle with prolotherapy. Since this was Craig's first sprain, I did not want to do so.

I explained to them that when you sprain your ankle for the first time when you are fourteen years old, in a few weeks your ankle injury most often heals up naturally. You do your exercises, wear your brace, and go back to playing basketball. Later, if Craig showed any sign of symptomatic ankle instability, that is when I would recommend prolotherapy.

If I am treating an athlete with whom I have worked before in both the old and new paradigm, then I might go right to RIT. This was the case with Ashleigh, then a nineteen-year-old, elite collegiate tennis player who, like Craig, also came in with a moderate ankle sprain. Ashleigh had first sprained her ankle when she was ten. She had gone through several rounds of conservative treatment and still had a somewhat unstable ankle. I had treated her a few years back with prolotherapy, and her ankle was doing well until she twisted it again in a match. She came in the next day, and because of her past treatment history we decided to try prolotherapy, something I had rarely done before on a new sprain. Ashleigh later reported that her ankle was still sore and swollen on the day of treatment, but the swelling was much better the following day. Within four days, she was in physical therapy, and a few days later, was out playing again.

Athletes like Ashleigh are the willing pioneers, always wanting to try cutting-edge care, thus paving the way for more widespread use of RIT.

Ashleigh still has unstable ankles because she has a genetic ligamentous laxity condition called Ehlers-Danlos syndrome, and they require consistent care while she continues playing tennis. I can tighten them up for a time, but I cannot get rid of the genetic predisposition of the ligaments to loosen back up like the rest of her ligaments. Ashleigh also has a bit of needle phobia, so even though she knows how well that prolotherapy treatment worked, she will sometimes sprain her ankle and go right to physical therapy, hoping to avoid injections.

"Whenever I tried to let my ankle heal on its own, it would not, and I would end up back for prolotherapy. With it, I could do PT in a few days and get back out to the court within a week. Sometimes I would go right from prolo to playing. The first twenty-four hours after a prolotherapy treatment could be rough, but it got easier as I had more treatments. Once I had both ankles treated at once, and that was harder, but I needed to get back to the court. My ankles are pretty good now, and I usually only need tune-ups every three or four months. I can tell when I need them. I see no cons to this treatment; only pros. I tell people to just go for it."

Athletes like Ashleigh are the willing pioneers, always wanting to try cutting-edge care, thus paving the way for more widespread use of RIT.

"DON'T TELL ME I HAVE TO STOP"

Of the many athletes I've treated over the years, some of the most challenging to keep going were the professional body builders. I have worked with men who were at the Mr. Universe level in the sport, and women competing in the Miss Fitness USA competition. They would literally come in and say, "Doc, do your thing. I have another injury, and I want you to fix it with prolotherapy." Earlier in my RIT work, when these athletes were younger and more actively competing, they would tell each other about these treatments, and it seemed as if I were taking care of an entire gym.

Many of these original patients are now retired from that sport, something that usually happens by forty years of age. One of my original female bodybuilders, Bridget, competed in the Miss Fitness USA competitions where she had to do a gymnastic routine as well as a body builder's pose on stage. Before she started seeing me, Bridget told me she wasn't being routinely treated for her injuries. Her doctor would give her painkillers when they proved absolutely necessary, and she had been to an orthopedic surgeon to have arthroscopic surgery on her right knee. The first thing she said to me was, "Don't tell me I have to stop." I never did. I treated her for fifteen different injuries over the years, most often with prolotherapy, but a couple of times with PRP. I also used old-paradigm treatments, like occasional cortisone shots, when they seemed indicated to try to get her through an impending competition.

She first came to me with a hamstring tendon injury that never completely healed. It never healed for two reasons. First, she needed to keep doing flying splits on stage for her gymnastics routine. Second, it is very common for this injury not to heal fully, regardless of the treatment employed. Hamstring tears are hard to heal, especially when they are high up, close to the bone. With high hamstring tears, PRP is my treatment of choice. I was able to help Bridget with her injury, but she, like some of the other patients I have treated for this injury, still had a nagging pain that never went away. I have had about a 75 percent success rate with helping heal high hamstring tears, which is much better than the surgical outcomes with which I am familiar.

I had greater success with some of Bridget's other recurring injuries. When I first treated the complete tear of the ulnar collateral ligament in her thumb, it completely healed with a couple of prolotherapy injections. Then, in a competition, she injured it again. Fortunately, a few more prolo treatments brought it back to normal. Later, Bridget tore the medial meniscus in her knee, and I treated it with PRP, which kept her going for a while. Then she reinjured it and had surgery. That worked until she tore it again. At that point, we used prolo to calm it down.

"Besides seeing you for RIT treatments," she reported, "I go to a massage therapist once a week and a chiropractor twice a week, but I'm not a big holistic person. I have no patience. I want instant results. I trust whatever treatment you suggest. I would recommend this treatment to anybody. The worst thing that can happen is you have an injection that doesn't work. I don't experience much pain with these injections. On a scale of five, it would be one and a half or a two, even with the PRP.

"I would alter my training after treatments, but I never stopped. I just trained right through the pain. I'm one of those serious athletes who gets the injections and then goes right to the gym. RIT didn't heal me 100 percent, but it enabled me to train and continue competing, and that is what I wanted. If it wasn't for the regenerative injection treatments, I never would have gotten as far as I did."

Bridget ranked among the top five female bodybuilders in the world during her career as a Miss Fitness USA Champion.

Another of my patients, Vinnie, is a good friend of Bridget. I've taken care of him for over ten years. I did a lot of prolotherapy on him, treating his elbow, knees, shoulders, feet, and wrist. I kept him competing until he was very high up in the sport. He relied on RIT as his go-to therapy. When he got injured, I would squeeze him in and get him well enough to keep going. Now that he is retired from bodybuilding, he is seriously involved with baseball and doing very well with it. He attributes part of his continuing success to the RIT treatments I did for him.

BACK IN THE GAME

In terms of frequent injuries, football players rank right up there with bodybuilders. One of the things that brought me to RIT was that I was looking for a better way to treat my own residual injuries from playing high school football.

Over the years, I have treated a number of professional, semi-professional, high school, and college players for a wide variety of injuries. Steven was a lineman for the Washington Redskins. He had suffered serious shoulder injuries over his seven-year career as a starting lineman in the NFL, and his cartilage was destroyed. His MRI showed advanced arthritis that was threatening to end his career. His doctors were telling him that he would have to have his shoulder replaced, which he was way too young to contemplate. He was referred to me by his physician and by his physical therapist, who specialized in myofascial release work.

Because of the severity of his injury, we went right to adult autologous stem cell injection treatment (ASCI). As his shoulder was recovering from the treatment, he did a lot with physical therapy and myofascial work. He was able to achieve excellent range of motion and strength, as well as pain relief. His team had released him because of his injuries, but his team's replacement wasn't doing such a great job. Steven had recovered so well that he was given another chance at returning to his former position. According to his physician, he had his best season ever.

I also treated Omar, an NFL player with the Denver Broncos. He had bilateral plantar fasciosis that was very resistant to treatment. He was actually seeing another prolotherapist at one point, without success. I performed one treatment on his right foot and two on his left, and he was able to play a complete season the next year. He came back to me the following season, after he had ruptured his patella tendon and had it surgically repaired. He ended up with chronic patella tendon pain. Two PRP treatments fixed that, and he was back to competing as a starting kickoff return specialist in the NFL.

Cory became my patient the summer before his senior year of high school. He was one of the outstanding quarterbacks in his county. He had torn his labrum playing volleyball at a party. A labral tear is very difficult to treat successfully, even with surgery. He was told by two well-known orthopedic surgeons in our area that he needed surgery and would miss his senior season. He and his family came to me with a stack of MRIs and x-rays and asked if I could help him. I saw Cory in July. We agreed to try PRP and follow it with prolotherapy. I did the first treatment about four weeks before practice started. I prescribed physical therapy to begin during week two of the treatment cycle, and I asked him to continue therapy through the first two weeks of practice, when his team would start playing scrimmages.

About six weeks after the PRP treatment, he came in and told me his shoulder didn't hurt, but he had problems throwing more than thirty-five yards. His shoulder felt loose and weak. In spite of the PT work, his shoulder was still unstable. He was not a candidate for surgery, and he would have lost the season if he had gone that route. I told him I could do more PRP, but that he could be out for two to four weeks and miss the first three games. He did not like that option, so I told him I could try prolotherapy. He would need to rest five days, but he could be back in the game the next weekend. He said, "That sounds great, let's do it." He called me after the second game and said, "My shoulder feels the best it has felt in my entire high school career. I'm throwing sixty-five yard bullets without a problem. I have no pain, and my arm is stronger than it has ever been."

The next game, he got thrown to the ground and reinjured his shoulder. So he came in and I treated him with prolotherapy one more time. After that, he reported that his shoulder was not perfect, but was strong. He was throwing well—so well he made all-county. He played basketball and baseball also that year, and ended up having a number of colleges trying to recruit him for their football programs. I continued treating him for other in-

---

"I would like to travel around doing a sales pitch to college athletic departments about RIT. I believe it is so much better than surgery."

---

juries he suffered playing both as a wide receiver and a wild cat quarterback for his college football team.

"I would have no problems coming to you for anything the rest of my life," he told me. "Sure, pain was an issue for about a week with PRP and for about three days with prolo, but these treatments gave me the chance to do something I love to do, both in high school and college. I always tell everyone about it. I think so much of it that I would like to travel around doing a sales pitch to college athletic departments about RIT. I believe it is so much better than surgery."

WORK YOUR WAY THROUGH IT

You don't have to be a bodybuilder or football player to sustain an injury. Jerome is involved in gym workouts and basketball during the week, and snow skiing and jet skiing on weekends. He was a passenger on a wave runner when he was rolled off it. In his right knee, the medial collateral ligament (MCL) snapped, the anterior cruciate ligament (ACL) was damaged, and there was a meniscal tear. Almost thirty years earlier, he had had part of his medial meniscus removed in a surgical procedure because he had a tear that could not be repaired at that time. Twenty years after that, he had torn his MCL playing tennis, causing him to give up the sport. Consequently, a good part of his MCL had remained intact, but he had a complete tear now. According to the MRI report, they could not rule out a complete tear of his ACL, but when I tested it clinically, the ACL seemed to be partially intact.

Because of the severity of Jerome's injury and his previous treatments, we decided to go directly to PRP. I injected what was left of his ACL, along with his MCL, and put him in a knee-stabilizing brace. As I have explained, RIT can only work on the ACL ligament if some of it is left. Following the PRP treatment, Jerome reported that he only needed a few doses of pain medication the day of the procedure and the morning after, and one day of rest. He was able to walk and, shortly after, to return to mild workouts at the gym. However, he still felt his knee was unstable, so we did another PRP treatment. After that, Jerome reported being completely pain free unless he pivoted the wrong way. After his second treatment, the tear was no longer discernible. The ultrasound showed that the MCL was regenerating and clinically the ACL was improving.

Jerome told me he would advise a potential patient to "anticipate some pain, work your way through it and make sure you take charge of getting your stability back."

George is definitely an active person. He started playing basketball and baseball as a child, played through high school and college, and then, after college, transitioned to triathlons. He had his first problem with spondylolisthesis, a slipping of the vertebrae in his lumbar region, in his early teen years. It probably stemmed from the repetitive, sometimes aggressive motions and odd angles necessary to play baseball. His doctor advised bed rest and told him to stay away from sports until it healed. George reported that, despite following his doctor's suggestions, it never really healed. He often had to take as much as six weeks off from sports when his back bothered him. The older he got, the more often it bothered him, and the worse the pain was. Core stability exercises helped but didn't solve the problem. Competing in triathlons exacerbated his condition and immobilized him for long periods of time. His doctor confirmed his problems all stemmed from spondylolisthesis, and recommended that George come to see me.

I did a series of radiological studies and determined that there could be some benefit from RIT treatment. Because this was a serious, longstanding condition that met the criteria for surgery, I recommended we use a combination of prolotherapy and PRP. The x-rays showed gross spinal instability in his lower spine of 4 millimeters of movement between flexion and extension x-ray views. Normally, there should not be any. A case is determined to need surgical fusion when the instability distance reaches 3 millimeters.

After two treatments, I ordered repeat x-rays and the measurement had decreased to 1 millimeter! This was an unexpected result, but one that I was elated to share with him. I gave him two more treatments about a month apart. He reported that within the first month, he felt a difference. "One thing is clear," George told me, "this works. It gave me this amazing feeling to discover there was a non-surgical approach that could do so much."

After the initial series of treatments, George felt better than he remembered feeling since his initial injury. I give him tune-ups on his lower back as needed, and I have treated him for five un-

---

"You could have prolotherapy during a training season and not miss a beat. I'm older, in my thirties, but I feel like I'm in my twenties. I feel like I have my youth back."

---

related injuries since then, including a neuroma in his foot, that resolved within two weeks. I treated minor tears in his shoulders and had him back to his normal activities within three days. He developed chronic pain in his ankles due to recurrent sprains and has had four treatments done on his left one. Now that his left ankle has healed, I'll work on the right one to help return both his ankles to stable, pain-free function.

George still competes in amateur triathlons and attributes his ability to do these intense races to the RIT treatments he has received. He characterizes his recovery as fast. "I was mobile, I could do things, but I couldn't move quickly. Everything was done at a turtle's pace, but I still went back to work the same day. You could have prolotherapy during a training season and not miss a beat. I'm older, in my thirties, but I feel like I'm in my twenties. I feel like I have my youth back. I would recommend that potential patients go in with a little faith and an open mind."

KEEP RUNNING WITH PROLOTHERAPY

Leah was in her mid-forties when she began running marathons. Prior to that time, she had been involved with women's basketball and with running five-kilometer and ten-kilometer races. A friend decided to try marathon running, and Leah thought she would give it a try with her. She loved it. She qualified for the Boston Marathon, completed it with a decent time, and then decided to run the Marine Corps Marathon. It was in this race that she tore the hamstring in her right leg. Despite the tear, she finished the race. She went to an orthopedist who told her she should stop running marathons. She did not like that advice, so she went to a variety of physical therapists, a few of whom did help her, but could not heal the tear. One of them suggested she see me.

From her diagnostic ultrasound scan, I could see there was scar tissue, and that her tear had healed itself up to a point, but not completely. I recommended she see a chiropractor who works with ART, and that gave her additional relief. But it was clear she would also benefit from prolotherapy. She researched it online and felt sufficiently reassured to give it a try. She did not find the treatments painful, and she was able to get back to some running within five to seven days after each treatment. Since her initial series of six treatments, she has seen me about four times a year for tune-ups, and comes in if she sustains any other injury from running.

"After the initial treatments," she told me, "I run as much or more than I did before, over greater distances, but not as fast. My advice to people is to try it. It's not very invasive, and there are no side effects. I just wish insurance would cover it."

The sole treatment I used with Leah was prolotherapy. Another runner patient also had an amazing outcome with prolotherapy. An Olympic runner, he competed in the 2012 London Games. He came to me with a calcification and chronic tear of his posterior tibial tendon, and I gave him a few prolotherapy treatments. He ran in a pool for a few days to give himself time to heal. According to his report and my ultrasound diagnosis, he did heal the tear completely, but the calcification persisted. Because of the great results he had with this treatment, he has referred me quite a number of people involved with track and field. One of them came in and told me, "He said you are the reason why he's still running." It is interesting that RIT is recognized as a legitimate treatment by many of the governing bodies in the Olympic sports community.

Natalie, a long distance runner from Pittsburgh, came to me because she had badly diseased bilateral Achilles tendons. Despite her pain, she raced all the time I was treating her. She could do so because she opted to only treat with prolotherapy. This allowed her to get treated on a Monday, cross train for a couple of days, then go back to running. It took Natalie about fourteen months of prolotherapy treatment, but she finally healed up. She knew that with another kind of RIT she could have healed more quickly, but she would have had to stop running for a longer time after each treatment. With PRP, she would have been out for a couple of weeks, and with ASCI, she could have been out for six weeks. Running was too important to her physical, emotional, and social life for her to want to stop training for those longer periods.

RUNNING ALL NIGHT

Brandon is an ultrarunner. This means he sometimes runs for more than one hundred miles straight, or for over twenty-four hours. Brandon has been running since he was twelve. He ran his first marathon when he was a senior in high school. He has run in the Boston Marathon, the New York Marathon, and the Marine Corps Marathon. From there he began doing some triathlons and Ironman competitions. He became fascinated with what his body could do and turned to ultrarunning, beginning with a run up and down Pike's Peak in Colorado. From there he ran in fifty-mile races and worked up to one hundred miles. He finished in the top ten in his first one hundred-miler, and told me, "I was hooked after that. Eventually, I tried a twenty-four-hour race, and discovered I'm actually better at those. It is really electric to be able to see the sun travel across the sky and be in the midst of this intense physical activity all day, then run all night. My goal is to run the Badwater Ultramarathon, a 135-mile race in Death Valley, California, in over-100-degree heat."

Brandon had a number of hamstring and other injuries over the years. What brought him to me was plantar fasciosis in his right foot and a medial meniscal tear in his left knee, injuries that occurred as a result of his first twenty-four-hour race. He told me he was running in mud and probably broke a piece of bone in his ankle or heel that tore the tendons in his foot. He kept running in that race and for a few weeks following. At that point, he twisted his knee because of the uneven gait he had developed, tearing his meniscus.

When I saw him, he wanted to go right to PRP for his knee. I agreed because of all his previous knee problems and the treatments he had had for them. In the first session, I treated his foot with prolotherapy and his knee with PRP. He swore his knee was fully working after that one injection, but we repeated the treatments again three months later, and he was very pleased with the results.

A few years later, he tore the meniscus in his right knee, and we treated that with PRP. "Look at my left knee now," he said during the treatment, "and you see a healthy knee. For me, that is a huge win-win. I expect the same will happen with my right knee. This running defines who I am as a person, and I'm not going to give it up. As long as PRP is working, there is no reason why I should change. PRP is so new people don't understand it. Even pro-football guys are like, 'What's that?' I think ten years from now it will be accepted. To me, it comes down to what is better for our overall health. I'd rather not have to use some kind of drug. I'd rather use PRP and all this other good stuff to keep me healthy. I hope it all becomes a mainstream thing sooner rather than later. If insurance covered it, then we would be heading in the right direction."

POWERFUL TOOLS FOR LIGAMENT INJURIES

Douglas was a twenty-two-year-old, Division I hockey player who played in Massachusetts. He injured his knee severely enough in a game that it required immediate surgery. While hospitalized, he contracted a joint infection with MRSA. The infection tore through his knee until he was missing half of the cartilage, and he developed an area of dead bone in the joint surface called an osteochondral defect (OCD). He required several surgeries during his four-week hospitalization. He had a fourth surgery called microfracture, in which the surgeon literally takes a sharp surgical tool and hammer to make pin holes in the dead bone. This is to stimulate bleeding and, hopefully, get stem cells to come out of the bone to create scar cartilage. This is meant for a much older player who is trying to get a few more years out of a seriously damaged joint. Unfortunately, the scar cartilage doesn't last, and in just a few years arthritis sets in. Douglas was suffering from chronic pain and recurrent effusions that needed to be drained every few weeks. After the microfracture surgery, he was still suffering the same symptoms, and playing hockey was out of the question. Douglas came to me not hoping to play hockey again, but rather just to be able to walk without a cane and maybe play with his own kids someday.

His tests showed he had a small tear in his anterior cruciate ligament (ACL) and a full-thickness grade-four osteochondral defect. That tear was so bad it looked like a mouse had taken a dime-sized chunk out of the weight-bearing section of Douglas's femur bone, and there was no cartilage around any of this section. There was significant swelling of the damaged bone, and he had a large joint effusion (fluid in the joint) as well. He elected to have a prolotherapy treatment over stem cells or PRP. I drained the fluid, injected his ACL, and did an intra-articular injection with 20-percent dextrose. It helped his pain and instability, and he showed few signs of fluid in his joint. He had another prolotherapy treatment when he returned six weeks later. Then he had a PRP treatment to see if we could initiate some healing of the cartilage six weeks after that.

I ordered a repeat MRI six months after his last treatment. Douglas's knee looked almost normal. The bone swelling was gone and the bone damage was over 90 percent healed. The ACL was completely normal. The cartilage showed over 50-percent healing. These are very difficult lesions to heal, even with the most sophisticated surgeries. Such operations can cost over

$50,000 dollars to perform and require extensive rehabilitation, repeat MRI scans, and bracing. Douglas is now able to play recreational ice hockey, as well as soccer. He plans to receive two PRP treatments a year. The hope is that continued periodic PRP treatments will help him grow his cartilage back to normal, so that he won't have to worry about a joint replacement until he's an old man. This case had such an excellent outcome that I presented it to a prolotherapy research conference in Madison, Wisconsin, at the Hackett-Hemwall Foundation.

There are many other great outcomes I see on a daily basis. These, while perhaps not quite so amazing as the one highlighted above, seem remarkable to the injured person who has only had experience with old-paradigm treatment. One of these was Jennifer, a high school volleyball player who was so good she had over a dozen colleges vying for her when she entered her senior year. In a game, she had sustained a soft tissue and bony Bankart lesion, damage to a very important labral cartilage complex in the bottom part of her shoulder joint. She was afraid this injury would end her volleyball career and her chance for an athletic scholarship. She'd been offered surgery that would have ended her volleyball season before it got underway, and with it, her chances for a scholarship. Her mother brought her to see me, and after two prolotherapy treatments, she was back to playing tournaments in front of the college scouts. We decided to do a PRP treatment before her winter travel season just to be sure her shoulder held up well while she played. It did, and she got the scholarship.

As these stories illustrate, both PRP and prolotherapy are powerful tools in helping ligaments that are partially torn. I have seen them work even on fully torn ligaments, such as those in the ankle and elbow, where the ligaments don't rupture and disappear like the ACL does. These other ligaments are still there even when they are completely torn, lying all stretched out. When you do RIT and proper physical therapy, those ligaments start to creep back and the fibers knit back together again. Before you know it, you have a normal ligament that you can accurately image using diagnostic ultrasound or MRI.

HELPING TENDON TROUBLES

RIT is equally helpful in tendon injuries. One of the most common of these is what is frequently called "tennis elbow." The common extensor tendon is what usually tears, although this injury can also be caused by an unstable joint with a ligament tear, compounded by tendinitis, or small tears or calcification in the tendons.

Gina's case is an example of how I now typically treat tennis elbow with RIT. She was a competitive tennis player with chronic pain in her elbow. I treated her with prolotherapy. After the first treatment, she had severe pain that lasted about three or four days. By day five, she was back to her baseline, and by day seven, she was starting to feel some relief. With each treatment, she got better and had much less pain. After the second treatment, she was able to train and play some tennis using an elbow strap. At the end of four treatments, she was 100 percent better.

Since I began using PRP for tennis elbow, I also have had good results with that treatment. Seth had gotten some relief with prolotherapy, but wasn't where he wanted to be. I suggested he try PRP, but warned him he might experience more significant pain than he had with prolotherapy. I had just been trained on my new equipment for making bloodless PRP and offered him the option to try it, explaining it might be less painful. He agreed, and we proceeded. Seth called me the next day to say, "Something's wrong with my elbow." I called him back to see what was wrong, and he said he had no pain. I had him come in and took a look. Everything was progressing as it should. I concluded that, at least for him, bloodless PRP works well and causes a significant reduction in pain. I ended up doing one more treatment with the bloodless PRP, and he was cured. The interesting part of his story is the anticipated post-procedure pain was non-existent. Although I expect less pain with bloodless PRP, his result is uncommon. When I see this outcome after a bloodless PRP treatment, I call that patient pretty darn lucky.

I have also had success with RIT for golfer's elbow. While tennis elbow involves the tendons and, commonly, the collateral ligament on the outside of the elbow, golfer's elbow involves the four tendons and, very commonly, the collateral ligament on the inside. These are normally harder to heal than the four outside tendons. Luke, a senior businessman I had treated for a knee injury, referred Jared, his golfing buddy, to me because Jared was suffering from golfer's elbow. After three PRP treatments, Jared was back to golfing with no pain or problem.

While my athlete patients are quick to try anything new, over time many of my other patients have decided to try the new healing paradigm. Some of their results have been as remarkable as those of the athletes described in this chapter. A major difference between athletes and the average Joe is that the athletes are more likely to come in when their injury is newer. Dealing with an acute injury gives a better opportunity for complete healing. Non-athletes often try self-care and old-paradigm care before they see me. Consequently, I often don't have the opportunity to treat them until their injury has become chronic.

CHAPTER TWELVE
TREATING CHRONIC INJURIES AND DEGENERATIVE DISEASES WITH THE NEW TREATMENT PARADIGM

Since the medical definition of a chronic injury is any injury that has not healed in six weeks, the majority of my patients would have injuries that fall into that category. If you have not received the appropriate care when you suffered an acute injury, if you have not followed through with the PRICES method of home care—discussed in Chapter Four—and/or physical therapy, or if you are over twenty-five years old, there is a high risk that most injuries will take more than six weeks to heal. Think about the athletes whose stories I shared in the preceding chapter. Even with the best of old-paradigm care, most of them ended up with chronic injuries. Non-athletes who are injured rarely treat acute injuries as aggressively as athletes do, so their acute injuries often become chronic.

When you enter the chronic injury category, the treatment you choose will greatly determine how good an outcome you can expect. Remember that a poorly treated chronic injury can often lead to reflex inhibition, which affects key muscles around the injured limb. Without the right kind of treatment, you could be headed toward dynamic stabilization failure, which affects the joints and muscles above or below the injury.

I have taken care to explain the old and new treatment paradigms in detail because I have seen so many patients who did not

---

Non-athletes who are injured rarely treat acute injuries as aggressively as athletes do, so their acute injuries often become chronic.

---

receive proper treatment at the initial stage of their injury end up with either lingering pain or a degenerative condition. There are so many ways this can happen. A common one is the athlete who is willing to play through his or her initial pain. But there are many others. In this chapter, I will recount some stories of people I have treated whose injuries progressed from acute to chronic, and sometimes to degenerative. I will let them tell you about the treatment they received from doctors following the old paradigm and about the new-paradigm methods that were able to give them some relief.

"NO SERIOUS INJURIES"

Sean is an active man in his late sixties. He is retired from his executive position with a major company, but keeps busy with remodeling projects both for himself and for his church. He is also a hiker who once hiked the Appalachian Trail, and was used to taking twenty-mile hikes until he was injured. Sean was repairing the roof on his historic home when a tile came loose under his foot, and he fell over twenty feet. When he told me his story, he emphasized that he "escaped serious injury." He did, however, have quite a number of resultant problems I found grim. After his fall, his daughter had driven him to the emergency room where they diagnosed him with a broken arm, rotator cuff tears, an injured neck, a sprained sacroiliac (SI) joint, and an extremely severe sprain of his left foot. Despite all of these injuries, they treated him only in the emergency room and sent him home with braces, crutches, pain medication, and instructions to contact his family physician. The radiologist called later and told Sean he had multiple, severe fractures of his calcaneus or heel bone.

Sean reported that the sacroiliac injury was the most painful initially because the nerves around the joint had been damaged. He went to an orthopedic surgeon who suggested fusing the SI joint. Sean declined, realizing that would adversely affect him for the rest of his life. That doctor sent him to a sports medicine specialist who treated him with manipulation. This helped some, but not enough. The SI pain became a chronic problem, which no one seemed to be able to help. Sean was getting regular epidurals to block the pain. He had a bad experience with one of them. The doctor hit a nerve and paralyzed him for a few minutes. One of the sports medicine docs he was seeing recommended he consult with me, adding that I used "unconventional methods, but they worked." This was two years after Sean's original fall.

Using manipulation, I was able to set Sean's SI joint, which gave him some relief. I did give him some cortisone shots initially because he had such severe sciatic pain it once caused him to pass out. After a few adjustments, I suggested we add prolotherapy. Sean agreed, and his back pain is now cured as a result of prolotherapy and manipulation. In fact, he told me after the initial set of treatments, "I have never had another problem with my SI joint or spine. I am back to 100 percent there." Sean still had quite a number of other issues.

When I got his back under control, I began working on his shoulder with prolotherapy. That was a slower and more painful process for Sean, but we made good progress, and he now reports his shoulder is 100 percent better.

"You do not get instant results," Sean said. "But if this can eliminate surgery, I would not do it any other way. When I had rotator cuff surgery, it took over a year to heal. This is much different. I didn't have the pain of surgery or six weeks of immobilization. I feel this is definitely a viable alternative for a lot of things."

The most difficult problem we had to resolve was with Sean's heel bone, or calcaneus. When he first injured himself, he had been treated by a prominent orthopedic foot surgeon at one of the well-known teaching hospitals in Philadelphia. After Sean's third unsuccessful surgery to repair the calcaneus fracture and a damaged tendon, the surgeon said she wanted to reconstruct it. He did not want this. "I had been through enough pain and trouble," he told me. He asked me to see what I could do. Using high-resolution ultrasound, I was able to make an accurate diagnosis. I found that the surgeon, while trying to repair a chronic fracture in the calcaneous, had inadvertently screwed the sural nerve into the calcaneus bone. I had to use a neurolysis treatment, which is injecting a severely injured nerve with a 4-percent phenol solution that kills the nerve and thus relieves the pain.

Then I used prolotherapy to take care of a tear in his peroneal tendon, and while I was in there, I shaved down several bone spurs with a large needle. The bone spurs developed near the screw holes where his surgical hardware had been placed during one of his surgeries. These spurs had kept Sean from being able to do physical therapy. They would irritate his damaged nerve, which had been rubbing against two of the screws the surgeon had used to repair his heel bone fracture. After he recovered from these treatments, Sean noted most of his pain was gone.

Sean reports he can now walk three miles a day, and is back at the gym working out with weights. His goal is to be able to resume the twenty-mile hikes he used to enjoy taking. However, he is very satisfied with his pain relief and increased function. Before ultrasound-guided prolotherapy, percutaneous cheilectomy (bone spur removal) and neurolysis were used, a patient like Sean—and there are more than you would think—would only have had the options of further exploratory surgery or lifelong pain management.

LIFE CAN CHANGE IN AN INSTANT

As a girl and young woman, Lucille was a gymnast. When she was ten, she developed a knee problem called Osgood-Schlatter's disease, which is an irritation of the growth center, where the patella tendon (kneecap tendon) attaches to the upper shin bone or tibial tuberosity. Her right knee would swell when she did her gymnastic routines. The doctor ordered her leg to be in a cast for six weeks, which was then a not-so-common treatment for that condition. Her leg didn't swell again. However, her condition made the attachment of her patella tendon at the tibial tuberosity enlarge, so it appeared as a bigger than normal bump of bone over her upper shin where the patella tendon attaches. This would sometimes cause her pain.

Nonetheless, she had lived a very active lifestyle. She hiked, swam, skied, biked, and did both yoga, and Zumba. A few years back, she went roller skating with her family. She fell and hit her right knee right on the tibial tuberosity, causing the enlarged bone to fracture. She had surgery to remove the fractured piece of bone from her upper shin bone, and that is when her real problems began.

The doctor she saw sent her for physical therapy at a level usually reserved for professional athletes. I can only surmise he heard she had been a gymnast and assumed she was still at that level of activity. Lucille was in constant, severe pain. She went to the head of sports medicine at one of the Philadelphia hospitals, and he said he had no idea how to help. He sent her to the pain management program at a respected rehabilitation facility. She went three days a week for three hours, doing aqua therapy, regular physical therapy, isometrics, and massage. She was making some progress, but still had debilitating pain. One of the doctors there referred her to me.

When I first saw Lucille, two years after her fall, she had been in daily pain for all of that time. She had been diagnosed as having reflex sympathetic dystrophy in her right leg, a condition that is now being called chronic regional pain syndrome (CRPS) type 1. She had needed daily pain medication. She could barely bend her knee and walked with a pronounced limp. She was unable to drive or do much in the way of caring for her three young children. Her entire family had been profoundly affected by the injury. She believed she would have this as a lifelong problem.

When I first performed a diagnostic ultrasound on the day of her initial evaluation, I discovered she had a patellar tendon tear that was definitely contributing to her pain. It had gone undetected. It could have been a result of the fall, and remained undiscovered by the surgeon, who assumed her pain was coming from the fractured piece of bone. It could also have been caused by the aggressive physical therapy she initially performed. Since then, Lucille had continued doing physical therapy on a constant basis, and it had exacerbated this underlying problem. I realized she needed to calm down the pain to get rid of the reflex inhibition and dynamic stabilization failure that were contributing to her misery. I had her stop physical therapy and rest. She rested her knee for over a year while I treated the pain and the underlying tendon problems.

The first thing I noticed before I treated Lucille was her surgery scar was red and inflamed. She still had pieces of suture material inside the scar. She had noticed pieces of suture had worked their way to the surface of the skin over the two years since the surgery. When I treated her the first time, I numbed her scar with lidocaine and used a scalpel and tweezers to remove several more pieces of suture from her scar. I then did several perineural superficial injections, and after the first few, her scar was skin-colored and no longer chronically inflamed. This was an important aspect of cleaning up her nerve pain, because chronic scar pain acts as an interference field in the network of nerves that are irritated in a CRPS patient. Once that interference field is normalized, the nervous system can begin to heal.

I then began treating Lucille with PSI every two weeks to calm down her chronic nerve pain from the CRPS type 1. I encouraged Lucille to get a home-use ultrasound machine, which can be used to drive dextrose mixed in ultrasound gel underneath the skin where the nerves lie, and thus provide some relief between treatments. When the nerve pain improved, Lucille had five PRP treatments, four months apart.

Her early treatments were very painful, but she experienced

significant pain relief for a while after each. The CRPS type 1 went away at a couple points during her course of PSI, but it came back after she reinjured her knee in the middle of treatment. The last PRP was a bloodless one, which noticeably diminished her post-treatment discomfort. Her recovery was also much quicker. As she improved, she added acupuncture, massage, and yoga to her treatment. She needed hormone replacement therapy because chronic pain medication plays havoc with the body's hormones.

"It has been a long road," Lucille recounted. "But I believe I can be healed. I don't walk with a limp anymore, and I am able to bend my knee. I used to have lots of holes in my patellar tendon. Now I only have one small one left. RIT is cutting-edge technology. And what has really helped is your bedside manner, which is the best of any doctor I have ever gone to. You really care and have a true relationship with your patients. One time, I asked you what would have happened to me if I had not found you and this treatment. You told me I would have had to use a cane, and probably would have been in a wheelchair. For a thirty-something mother of three little kids, that was a pretty frightening thought."

Peter had suffered an infection as a child that had necessitated the amputation of his left arm. That had not stopped him from founding and running a successful farm. While he was lifting himself out of an unfinished half basement, he suffered a full-thickness tear of his rotator cuff tendon in his right shoulder. He saw an orthopedic surgeon, who suggested an operation. He cautioned Peter that he would not be able to use that arm for six weeks to six months while it healed. Peter was afraid his business could go under in that amount of time. He had heard about my work from a friend, and came to see what I could offer. Considering his circumstances, I felt PRP with a fat graft would be the best way to go. He agreed, and after his first treatment, he only lost four days of work. After the second, he only lost three, and those two treatments were enough to repair his tendon. We had been able to schedule the PRP on Friday, so he would lose as few work days as possible. Peter was soon back to his farm, and his business continued successfully.

RELIEF DID COME

Mae had been in a horseback accident when she was ten years old. She had been thrown by a horse and landed on her neck and shoulders. At that time, few people used helmets. Mae ended up with a broken collarbone and a seriously injured neck. Shortly after the accident, she began to get migraine headaches. They were an almost daily occurrence. She went to doctor after doctor, and eventually had surgery to repair some of the damage to her shoulder. That helped her shoulder pain, but did nothing for her headaches. She shared that many of the doctors she'd seen had told her there was nothing wrong with her.

Mae found a chiropractor who provided some relief, but she did not have the spinal stability to hold the neck adjustments. It was that chiropractor who suggested she see me. "You were the first doctor who listened to me," she said of our first meeting. "You looked at the anatomy of my neck and found where the problems were."

I suggested Mae try prolotherapy. She had treatments on her neck every six weeks for a year. By the end of that time, she had a lot more stability and the headaches had subsided. She could then go about six months between tune-up treatments. However, she still would get migraines.

She went to a neurologist who suggested medication. She went to a massage therapist, a physical therapist, and a cranial sacral specialist. Most of these treatments just exacerbated the migraines. We recently tried a form of PRP on her neck. This had good initial results.

"I will always appreciate that you validated that something was wrong," Mae told me. "With you, I always felt there was hope. My headaches, neck pain, and back pain are better, and so is my quality of life. If I get a headache that won't go away, you fit me in to get some perineural superficial injections, and they usually bring me back to baseline within a few days. I absolutely would recommend these treatments to anyone in my position who is wandering around wondering what is wrong with them. The pain and discomfort of the treatment is worth it because relief does come."

POST-POLIO SYNDROME

Nancy is a woman in her late fifties who contracted polio during an epidemic when she was an infant. This left her with a wide range of musculoskeletal problems, which over time resulted in her having four surgeries. These did little to help the dynamic stabilization failure stemming from the polio. As a result, one of her hip muscles, called the sartorius, ended up being surgically transferred to replace the quadriceps muscle that was rendered useless by the polio. She also developed tendinosis of the left iliopsoas muscle, the main hip flexor muscle, which crosses the hip joint. Nancy wears a brace from below her knee to her foot. She uses a cane as well. She gets ninety-minute massages every week. She gets chiropractic adjustments and Reiki, a form of energy healing. She told me she would not be able to walk without all of this.

Now a grandmother, Nancy has led an active work and social life, despite her physical problems. One day, she fell and landed on the already-injured hip. This caused her severe pain. She saw an orthopedic surgeon, who diagnosed her as having arthritis and suggested she have her hip replaced. She did, but it made no difference in her pain level. She described to me most of the doctors she had seen as being "in the box. By that, I mean they just try one medicine after another, and then physical therapy or surgery, and they ignore any and all new methods." Nancy was still working a forty-hour week, relying upon painkillers to get her through.

After suffering from chronic pain from the hip injury for a

"These treatments are on the cutting edge of what's happening, what's new, and what's working."

---

number of years, another physician suggested she see me. We tried a PRP treatment, although we both felt adult autologous stem cell injections would be most effective. At the time, Nancy did not have the financial means for ASCI. I tried several other methods to break up her scar tissue and give her more pain relief. One time, I was preparing to work on her scar tissue, and she felt an electric shock when I touched one area with a needle. Her reaction made me realize that when her tendon was surgically transferred to substitute for her quadriceps muscle, a nerve called the lateral femoral cutaneous nerve had been transferred with the muscle, and it became entrapped by the dense scar tissue in the front of her hip. So I ended up not doing the PRP we had planned on her scar tissue, but rather a hydrodissection of that nerve, in which I injected a large amount of dilute lidocaine between the scar tissue and the nerve to separate the nerve from the tissue entrapping it. A few days later, Nancy reported she felt the best she ever had since her fall.

During an appointment, Nancy told me that she would recommend other people to me "because of your confidence level. You weren't boastful, but you knew what you were doing and could explain it in layman's terms. You made me feel comfortable. You closed the lid on the box most of those other doctors are in, and just walked away. You are so far ahead of those guys that it's not even funny. These treatments are on the cutting edge of what's happening, what's new, and what's working."

SOMETIMES LATER IS BETTER THAN SOONER

Shannon was in her early fifties when her sedan was struck head on by a twelve-passenger van pulling out from a parking space onto the wrong side of the road. The impact was enough to cause major damage to her vehicle and injury to her. When cortisone shots and gentle physical therapy had calmed down the acute injuries, she still suffered with substantial rotator cuff pain and stiffness. Further physical therapy helped her regain some range of motion in her left arm and shoulder. The following winter, her car was again hit by a van. This accident exacerbated the initial damage to her rotator cuff.

Before seeing me, she had gone to an orthopedic surgeon who suggested arthroscopic surgery to see if cleaning out the area would help. He cautioned her, however, that due to the severity of the injuries and the arthritis in her shoulder, she would probably be looking at joint replacement surgery in the near future.

She came to me to see whether she might have any alternatives to that surgery. Because she had already exhausted the conservative treatments for her injury, we decided to try prolotherapy.

As can happen in the shoulder area, the initial prolotherapy treatment froze her shoulder for a time. This made her hesitant to continue. I suggested we try a long-acting numbing agent with a small amount of the prolotherapy solution. This gave her almost immediate pain relief. I carried out a series of such injections over several years. At that point, I told her about the success I had had with bloodless PRP, and she decided to try it. After the initial discomfort, she reported an improved range of motion and a significant reduction in the pain. While Shannon still had arthritis in the shoulder, she was now able to live with it.

With many types of arthritis, short of using stem cells, this is the best outcome I can offer patients at this time. Most of them realize that the longer they can put off replacement surgery, the better the surgical techniques and artificial joints will become, and they will realize a smaller chance of having revision surgery.

WHY ARTHRITIS IS REACHING
EPIDEMIC PROPORTIONS

I've already alluded to the fact that arthritis is almost an epidemic now, and the incidence of this disease is going to get worse. Three large contributing factors are that baby boomers want to keep doing the sports and activities they love, even when it hurts; obesity; and that children are becoming specialized in sports at an ever-younger age.

Ethan is a good example of the boomers. I spoke with him because he was considering the Regenexx method of stem cell treatment. He said other doctors had been telling him for a long time that he had arthritis of the knees. They also told him that continuing to run was beating up his joints, and one day soon, he would not be able to continue. He said, "They told me this day was coming, and now it is here. I can't believe it! I didn't think it was going to happen to me."

Luke shows what can happen to a youngster who specializes too early. A little leaguer since he could walk and throw a ball, Luke had hurt his pitching arm many times before he got to college. While playing for his team there, he fell on his right shoul-

> There is no free lunch when it comes to playing a sport that is going to further injure a joint.

der trying to catch a fly ball. He tore his labrum. When his doctor did radiologic tests, he saw that Luke already had signs of early arthritis. If he continues playing, he could be looking at replacement surgery before he is thirty. When I saw him for an evaluation, he was vehement about continuing to play. He was hoping to make it to the majors. In treating him with the new paradigm of care, we are both hoping for the best for him.

A question that patients commonly ask me is, "Does running (or pitching or bodybuilding or skiing, for example) cause arthritis?" The answer is no. There are seventy-year-old men and women who have pristine knees and run marathons. The key difference between these folks and a fifty-year-old who's running a marathon with arthritis of the knee is that the fifty-year-old had some kind of trauma to his knee when he was a young athlete in grade school or high school. Typically, the seventy-year-old long distance runner who has great knees never had an injury. Most likely, he didn't play sports, or at least contact and collision sports, when he was a young kid. If the individual is running pain free, the chances are good he'll be able to run for a long, long time without any problem, provided he takes good care of himself.

Another common question I get is, "If I have arthritis, will running (or another weight-bearing or contact sport) make my arthritis worse?" The answer is yes. If that person had a swollen joint at some point in his youth, or was injured and couldn't play for a week, chances are he is going to develop arthritis sometime earlier rather than later in his life. These patients should consider cross training or beginning to develop an interest in another sport that puts less pressure on weight-bearing joints. There is no free lunch when it comes to playing a sport that is going to further injure a joint. You are going to pay the price someday.

I never like to have the necessary conversation with my patients when they come in with bone-on-bone arthritis, asking, "When can I get back to marathon training?" That's a tough talk for patients and for me. They usually have not considered they would eventually have to hang up their running shoes and go do something else. After that talk, some patients would literally leave and never come back. They go look for someone who's going to give them more steroid shots so they can keep running. But steroid shots don't work forever. Others will come back with, "I'm not stopping, so you've got to fix me." I can't always do so.

I have a patient who is near sixty and an ultrarunner like Brandon. He works a full day and then runs for two or three hours every evening to prepare for ultramarathons. He admits he has beat-up knees, and he has done a lot of research about what his options are now and in the future. He knows one day it's going to catch up to him. But he has the money to pay for the best of new-paradigm treatments and the passion for the sport that will keep him running as long as he possibly can. If someone thoroughly knows the risks and is willing to suffer the consequences, that is his or her choice. For patients who don't realize the risks, I see my job as educator first, explaining the consequences of their activity and behavior. I am also their doctor, offering treatments that make sense medically, ethically, and financially, while helping them achieve their activity goals, both in the short term and long term.

I worry more about the people who don't do their homework and don't realize what arthritis can do to them in the future, both physically and financially. One example of the financial consequences is provided by Lily. Lily has chronic knee arthritis and no health insurance. Her passion is gardening, another activity that can be hard on the knees. She is a friend of one of my patients, who suggested she see me. Lily is on a limited budget, so I suggested we try treating her with prolotherapy. I see her about three or four times a year, and those treatments are enough to keep her moving, at least for now.

Could I help her more with PRP or stem cell therapy? I could, but she cannot afford those treatments. And she will certainly have a hard time affording the much larger cost of knee replacement when it comes to that point. Will Lily end up fairly immobile or in a wheelchair? I certainly hope not. Will she wait, like many patients, until Medicare can pay for her surgery? That could solve Lily's problem. But the huge number of people suffering from arthritis in the country is one of the factors that could break the Medicare bank.

Megan illustrates another sort of problem that can come with arthritis. She taught folk dancing until the arthritis in her hip forced her to have a hip replacement. The surgery did not go well, and she had a lot of complications that required her to have two revision surgeries before she was referred to me. After treating her for a time with prolotherapy to try to strengthen the ligaments and treat inflamed nerves around the hip, I wasn't seeing the results I expected. I sent her for further radiological studies, and it turned out her hip replacement was broken. She had to go for a third revision surgery. This time, following my advice, she made sure she was fitted with the proper type of replacement joint. She also went slowly and methodically through good physical therapy. Then I administered prolotherapy to tighten the ligaments around the hip and she did quite well. She is back teaching slow folk dances and letting her younger associates take care of the more energetic ones.

I see quite a number of people who have pain after a joint replacement. There are not too many conventional options open to them. After the surgeon has completed the replacement, he can't look at the area with an MRI because it is obscured by the metal joint. If he sends the patient for an x-ray, it usually looks fine because, unlike ultrasound, an x-ray does not show problems with tendons, ligaments, or entrapped nerves, nor does it indicate whether reflex inhibition or dynamic stabilization failure is present. These are foreign concepts to most surgeons anyway. So the surgeon tells the patient to keep trying physical therapy. If that doesn't work, the surgeon would most likely suggest the patient seek pain management. The patient who doesn't want to live with narcotic medications or with epidural injections or nerve block injections might find his way to a new-paradigm practitioner or an alternative practitioner who has other ways of dealing with the underlying problems.

I usually begin with these patients by doing an ultrasound diagnosis. Often I will see a big cyst, bursitis, or a tear. Sometimes the replacement hardware or the incision to put the hardware in has actually injured or trapped a nearby nerve. These are all things I can treat well using the appropriate old- or new-paradigm methods. Frequently, I can get rid of the pain, at least to some degree.

Recently, I've been doing more post-op, joint replacement referral work because there are a couple of orthopedic surgeons in my area who have sent me patients with chronic pain to see if I can help. I confer with the surgeons, telling them what I have found and what I would do. Some agree with my suggestions; others don't.

For post-operative pain, I have done a lot of PSI work, which helps ease the discomfort many of these patients are feeling. Sometimes this relief is permanent. Other times it is not. Half of those I've seen for post-operative pain have had to have their joints resized during a revision. Their joint replacement was too big or too small, or had loosened up. When they had the joint replacement revised, and followed that surgery up with new-paradigm care, many of these people were able to live life pain free.

Angie was one of these patients. Her husband was a physician's assistant who heard me speak and asked me if I could help his wife. She had suffered a fall on their vacation and severely injured her knee. The orthopedic surgeons in that area of the country told her she had to have a knee replacement immediately. After her joint replacement surgery, she did some physical therapy before returning home, but was still in pain. Upon examination,

I found that she had loose ligaments. When a knee joint is re-placed, two of four ligaments around the knee are removed, and the two remaining ones should be enough to stabilize the joint. Hers were not. I treated her once with prolotherapy to tighten the remaining ligaments, and a few days after treatment, her pain was significantly reduced, although she still wasn't feeling stable. Upon x-ray exam, it appeared that the joint replacement was too small. She went to a good orthopedic surgeon, and he agreed with my findings. So she had revision surgery, got the right size replacement, followed it up with good physical therapy and a few prolotherapy treatments, and is now doing very well.

Was her original problem arthritis in the knee that was ex-acerbated by her fall, or was it extremely loose ligaments, possi-bly sprained or torn by the fall? Did she actually need the joint replacement, or would RIT have fixed her? In an emergency, particularly in a place away from home, you often don't have the option to explore the situation thoroughly. But under normal circumstances, I always advise patients, particularly those with chronic or degenerative problems, to go to the doctor prepared. Know your options, have your questions ready, and be sure to get the answers before you proceed.

CHAPTER THIRTEEN
PREPARING FOR AND RECOVERING FROM AN RIT TREATMENT

If you asked one hundred of my patients about their RIT treatment, you would get one hundred different descriptions of the experience. Some of my patients feel little pain. Others are hypersensitive. A few people are quiet, many breathe deeply, some sigh, others have shouted. I've had some patients who wanted to watch everything. Many more keep their eyes closed. Some like to chat while others seem to be meditating. It is impossible to give a catchall description of what a treatment will be like because it is such an individual matter.

Reactions to the treatment also depend on the general health of the person having it, his activity level, where the injury is located, and his pain tolerance. Also relevant are the type of RIT a patient is having, and how many times he or she previously had it. For most people, PSI is the easiest treatment. While I might give a large number of injections during a single PSI treatment, they are superficial and really do feel like a series of little pinches to most people. The only exceptions to this would be when I am treating a person suffering from a disorder that makes him extremely sensitive to any touch.

Prolotherapy is definitely a bigger pinch. I have told you stories of people who had multiple reactions to it, from very small to very large. Usually, the first couple of treatments seem to cause a more intense response. People coming in for tune-up injections often have a minimal reaction. I've even had professional athletes go directly from the treatment to the gym, although I prefer that

---

It is impossible to give a catchall description of what a treatment will be like because it is such an individual matter.

---

people rest the treated area for at least that day. PRP requires both a blood draw and an injection into the injured area, so it can be more painful, especially if the PRP is red with blood. A blood-less PRP injection can be no more painful to receive than a pro-lotherapy treatment because the lack of red blood cells makes it much less irritating. ASCI, the longest and most complex procedure, can be painful both at the points of extraction and injection.

New research published by the Regenexx research lab showed it is safe to use lidocaine and preferably ropivicaine in very small doses (no more than 0.015 percent of lidocaine and 0.25 percent of ropivicaine) with a bone marrow concentrate injection. At this dose, the anesthetic will not harm the stem cells. If the dose is higher than this minimal effective level it will kill the stem cells outright. ASCI would seem like it would require the longest time for recuperation, but that is not necessarily so. Some post-AS-CI-treated patients have told me they took one pain pill, had one tough day, and by the next day, their pain was gone and never came back. Others have had more than three weeks of pain. In the first few days, these patients experienced severe pain, requiring bed rest, pain medication, and ice.

While all RIT treatments can cause such pain in some people, this is not normally the case. It depends on the person's pain tolerance, what I have to treat, how aggressively I have to treat it, and what part of the anatomy I am treating. It also depends upon how numb they become from the lidocaine injection, and how well the post-procedure pain medication works for them. However, the discomfort, potential complications, and downtime for all of these treatments is less than it would have been if a patient had undergone surgery.

The following are preparations I advise patients to make before undergoing any form of RIT. I urge patients to educate themselves about the procedure and be prepared well before the day of treatment. The amount of preparation coincides with the comprehensiveness of the treatment. Hence, there are few preparations for PSI, and many for ASCI. In this chapter, I first list the simplest preparations, and then I add the more extensive ones. If you have any questions not answered here, ask your doctor during the consultation before you even make the appointment for your RIT. Because RIT is constantly evolving, I am only going to tell you about the dos and don'ts I consider have sufficient scientific evidence backing them, or ones I have determined work well through my extensive practical experience at the time of writing. Your doctor might have others.

PREPARING FOR PSI

PSI is superficial injections of low-dose dextrose or dextrose with lidocaine administered to the nerves that lie just beneath the skin. It is theorized that PSI reduces the output of abnormal pathologic nerve protein molecules produced by inflamed nerves. It does so by blocking calcium channels in the nerve and allowing the nerve to return to a healthy normal state. Unlike the reaction in other forms of RIT, the dextrose used in PSI calms the nerve swelling down. It does not initiate a healing cascade. Consequently, NSAIDs and other drugs that interfere with other forms of RIT do not seem to do so with this treatment. As of the time of writing, we do not know of any particular regimen necessary to prepare for perineural superficial injection treatment.

PREPARING FOR PROLOTHERAPY

While prolotherapy treatments can differ greatly among individuals, and for the same individual on different occasions, the following are some suggestions to make your treatment most effective and comfortable.

1. Stop aspirin-containing medication seven days prior to your treatment. It is okay to continue taking baby aspirin unless told otherwise by your doctor. If you are on full-dose aspirin for a life-threatening condition, such as a deep vein thrombosis or a stent in a coronary artery, you must get written permission from the doctor who prescribed it prior to stopping your medication. This is very important.

2. Stop any other non-steroidal anti-inflammatory medications five days prior to your injection treatment.

3. With prior approval of your doctor, stop taking anti-platelet agents (Plavix, Ticlid) seven days prior to your injection.

4. With prior approval of your doctor, stop taking Coumadin (warfarin) five days prior to your injection. I require written clearance from your doctor before you stop, and a fax the

morning of your appointment showing your blood-clotting values (STAT PT, PTT, and INR) on that day.

5. If you smoke, stop. Having treated some smokers who quit during the course of their treatment, I have seen a difference in patients before and after they quit. While I cannot cite any scientific studies explaining why, nicotine is a potent vasoconstrictor. If your blood flow is constricted, then your body can't get blood to the diseased tissue as well as it would without nicotine in your system.

6. Be aware of the nutritional composition of the things you eat and drink, especially in the weeks before RIT. Optimal results can be improved with appropriate nutritional support. You should have a protein intake of at least 0.75 grams per pound of body weight. This means, for example, that a 125-pound woman should eat at least 94 grams of protein per day, and a 175-pound man should eat at least 131 grams of protein per day. Avoid foods that are known to increase inflammation, such as members of the nightshade family (peppers, tomatoes, potatoes, and eggplant).

7. Every day take:
   - A good multivitamin.
   - At least 50 milligrams of zinc.
   - One to two grams of vitamin C. Zinc and vitamin C are co-factors in the tissue-healing process.
   - A supplement that helps cartilage and stem cells grow (I recommend Ligagenix and/or Stem X Cell).
   - 1,500 milligrams per day of glucosamine.
   - 1,200 milligrams of chondroitin.
   - 50 milligrams of hyaluronic acid.
   - 500 milligrams of methylsulfonylmethane (MSM).

A product I recommend is Viosan Joint Health, which combines glucosamine, chondroitin, hyaluronic acid, and MSM. Take two each at breakfast and dinner if your joint was treated.

8. You may have a light meal prior to your RIT procedure. Avoid eating approximately two hours prior to the treatment.

9. It is highly recommended you have someone drive you home after your treatment, especially the first time, and always if you are using narcotic medication. After their initial few prolotherapy treatments, some patients who do not require medication are able to drive themselves.

AFTER INJECTION INSTRUCTIONS FOR PROLOTHERAPY

You have received an injection into several ligaments and/or tendons surrounding a joint, and possibly into the joint. As you know from reading *Regenerative Healing for Life*, the medication injected is designed to strengthen weak ligaments, heal damaged tendons, and/or treat arthritis pain. It does so by causing a local inflammatory reaction, which begins a tissue repair process. It is normal and expected to experience pain at the injection site for a few days. It is common after injections to have some swelling, particularly when the injection has been in the extremities. This swelling will usually go away in four to five days. You may take acetaminophen or a prescribed analgesic pain medication to decrease the pain.

1. Do not use any non-steroidal anti-inflammatory drugs such as naproxen, Celebrex, ibuprofen, or full-dose aspirin. Also do not use any steroid drugs, such as prednisone, during the course of your treatment. These drugs will stop or decrease

the beneficial effects of the treatment.

2. While it's not part of your treatment to heal your injury, you may ice the treatment area for pain relief during the first two days after the injections. Place an ice bag over the painful area up to ten minutes every thirty minutes to an hour, as needed, for pain control.

3. Optimal results can be improved with continuing the appropriate nutritional support and supplements listed above (see "Preparing for Prolotherapy").

4. It takes about three weeks for the body to achieve about 85 percent of the treatment effect. In general, injections are scheduled every three to six weeks to take advantage of your body's own natural healing powers.

5. Do not overuse the joint, tendon, or other treated body part. Sometimes this happens because a patient has a job that will not allow him to take enough time to rest. Other times it occurs because the patient is so anxious to get back to his gym or sport. Or the patient can be a parent of young children without sufficient backup help. I know it is difficult to find downtime, but frequently, a few days of rest could avoid years of chronic pain or more treatments than would otherwise be necessary to heal your injury.

6. If you are receiving manipulation treatments by an osteopath or chiropractor, ask him to avoid frequent, forceful, high-velocity methods until treatment is completed. High-velocity manipulation methods should be used sparingly (one to two times per month or fewer) after an injection treatment is performed.

7. Physical therapy, including myofascial release therapy, is recommended as soon as the pain is relieved (or nearly so)

and the stiffness and swelling are gone. *Caution*: Myofascial release and deep tissue massage can cause your treatment area to flare if done too early after treatment.

8. Get seven to eight hours of sleep and develop a positive outlook regarding your journey to full healing and recovery. Your mind and spirit are a powerful influence on your recovery.

ACTIVITY AFTER FIRST PROLOTHERAPY TREATMENT

Use the following as your guidelines for activity after treatment.

1. Begin stretching and strengthening exercises as instructed by your doctor. Be sure you are only extending at nearly pain-free angles and using force that does not cause more than mild discomfort. Continue targeted stretching and strengthening of your treated limb, at least until you're back to full activity.

2. When you are pain free, your physician or physical therapist may recommend additional stabilization exercises to reverse the reflex inhibition and to restore normal muscle firing patterns and biomechanical movement.

3. For the first five days after a treatment, do not do your usual workouts. Do the stretching and strengthening as described above. Do your normal activities of daily living as you are able. Take walks.

4. In the second week after your treatment, you can work out gently, use the pool, bike, or elliptical trainer. If you are a runner or triathlete, walk or jog as tolerated, beginning at a speed of eight or more minutes per mile. As you can tolerate it, increase your speed and distance, one at a time, not both at once, which could aggravate your healing injury.

5. In the third week after treatment, do aerobic, not anaerobic,

exercise. Increase your workouts, walk, or run, as fast as you can tolerate, but only in intervals of 100–200 meters.

6. Do not do eccentric workouts, in which you contract the muscle while lengthening it (as in a deep-knee squat), until your pain drops 80 percent or more. It is all right to do your workouts at 50–80 percent of normal until you reach this point in your recovery. If you experience an increase in your pain that does not go away for a day or two, your workout intensity is too high. You know your workout intensity is about right if, as a rule, after your workout, your pain returns back to its baseline within a few hours. If it stays elevated as described above, decrease your workout intensity to a previous level you tolerated for another two to three days, and then try to progress again.

7. In the fourth week after treatment, you can return to full, unrestricted activity as tolerated. If your injury is still painful, do not progress to the next level of activity until you are reevaluated by your physician.

ACTIVITY AFTER SECOND AND SUBSEQUENT PROLOTHERAPY TREATMENTS

You can add these guidelines to the ones above for subsequent treatments.

1. Stretch, strengthen, walk, and do activities of daily living for the first three days after treatment.
2. From the fourth day on, as tolerated, you can resume your exercise at whatever comfortable level you had previously reached, and progress from there.

ADDITIONAL PRE- AND POST-INJECTION INSTRUCTIONS FOR PRP

In addition to all the above instructions for prolotherapy treatment, you should also follow the instructions below if you have had a platelet-rich plasma (PRP) treatment.

1. You will be very sore about forty-five minutes after the treatment, particularly if the PRP was injected into a tendon. This can be a "something is definitely wrong" level of soreness. Take it easy the first few days.

2. Use acetaminophen tablets with codeine, one to two tablets every four to six hours, as needed, for pain. If your doctor has prescribed an alternative pain reliever, take that as prescribed. Stay ahead of the pain and don't wait for it to get too bad. These pills may make you drowsy or upset your stomach. Take them with food to help minimize the stomach upset. If they make you feel drowsy or loopy in the head, you should not drive or do any activity where you may hurt yourself or someone else.

3. If your administering physician also has prescribed stronger narcotic pain pills, only take them if you need to, and only take one type of medication at a time. If you need to take a stronger prescription medication, you must wait four hours after the dose of the other medication. These can definitely impair both mental speed and motor skills, and you must not drive or do any activity where you may hurt yourself or someone else. You may need these pills only at night, and only for the first one to three days, maximum. Don't use them if you don't need them. They will also constipate you, so increase the fiber in your diet, drink more water, and take a stool softener if needed.

4. After the first two to three days, the pain should lessen significantly. You will start having "good days and bad days," where you have more or less soreness. This is a good response, a sign your immune system is starting the healing process.

5. During your recovery period, keep track of your symptoms. Your doctor will discuss your progress with you when you return for your checkup.

6. See your doctor for reevaluation at four to eight weeks. Chronic conditions will likely take at least three treatments to reverse. If more injections are needed, they are usually performed every six to twelve weeks.

7. As per the instructions above concerning preparation for prolotherapy treatments, be aware of what you eat and drink, especially in the weeks before and after treatment. Remember to have sufficient protein intake, at least 0.75 grams per pound of body weight every day. Particularly when in healing mode, the body needs a good amount of protein, as well as a diet rich in nutrients. Adequate water is also critical. Avoiding smoking, excessive alcohol use, and the use of recreational drugs will also help the body to do the best job of healing.

8. In my fifteen years of performing RIT treatments on my patients, I have observed vegetarians seem to have a tougher time healing from their injuries than do non-vegetarians. I know of no study documenting this. However, other physicians practicing integrative orthopedic medicine have also observed this in their patients' healing outcomes. The difference usually manifests either as a less-than-optimal healing response, or in our needing to treat an injury more

times than we would expect. Also, when I have discussed this observation with patients, and they elect to change their diet to one with high-quality, lean animal protein of sufficient quantity, they usually heal more quickly. While this does not happen in all vegetarians, it happens with enough frequency that I believe patients should consider that vegetarianism may contribute to a poor injury-healing response before and after RIT.

9. You should continue taking at least a good multivitamin, and the other supplements listed above (see "Preparing for Prolotherapy").

ACTIVITY AFTER A PRP TREATMENT

It is critical that you follow the guidelines below after you receive PRP.

1. For the first two days, no activity, rest only. Use crutches for twenty-four hours if the treatment was on your legs or feet.

2. On day three, begin to move the limb/joint through its full range of motion without resistance. Move it around, try to return to a normal range of motion by holding the stretch your doctor has prescribed. Generally, you hold the stretch for thirty seconds, repeat three times per session, doing at least two to three sessions per day.

3. On day three, along with your range-of-motion sessions, it's okay to begin walking, swimming, and biking at low resistance if you can tolerate these activities. Do not overdo it.

4. On days ten to fourteen, begin doing the strengthening exercises as your doctor or physical therapist has instructed. Do two sets of ten to twenty gentle repetitions, twice per day. Gradually increase your resistance. It is vital to move

the limb to stimulate proper healing. Cross train for your cardio workout as you are able. Swimming, deep-water running, upper-body biking, recumbent biking, elliptical training, or walking can all provide good cardio workouts.

5. Runners, if a tendon in your leg or plantar fascia was injected, you can start jogging at four weeks if you feel at least 80 percent pain relief. If you have significant pain, or it takes a day or two to recover from a jog, stop and try again a few days later.

6. Formal physical therapy or a graduated home strengthening program can usually start at four to eight weeks, if you feel at least 80 percent recovered.

PREPARATIONS TO MAXIMIZE THE BENEFIT OF A STEM CELL TREATMENT

My associates at Regenexx and I are often asked how patients can improve the quality of their stem cells before a procedure in order to maximize the benefit of their treatment. The research is at a point where, with our combined experience of more than a decade, there are quite a number of guidelines we can give. Many of the guidelines in this section are adapted from the blog of Chris Centeno, M.D., one of the founders of Regenexx (visit www.Regenexx.com/blog).

1. **Cut the sugar.** We Americans consume way too much sugar. What do I mean by sugar? Not only the white granular stuff, but also bread, pasta, juice, super sweet fruits, and so on. All of this stimulates too much insulin production, which, combined with far too little activity, can cause metabolic syndrome. Consider going on a strict Atkins, Paleo, Zone, or South Beach diet. These are all low-glycemic diets, which

means that they can help control blood sugar and excessive insulin release. Ideally, you'll want to do this for at least one to three months before your procedure. Your physician should check your hemoglobin A1C (HBA1C) before and after you change your diet. It can take up to six months for the levels to fall. The Hemoglobin A1C value you're aiming for is 5.1. Another quicker test to see if you've beaten sugar addiction is what I call the "chocolate bar test." Get 70 percent, 80 percent, and 90 percent cacao bars and taste them. If you try the 70 percent bar and feel it's not sweet enough, go back to square one, you're a major sugar addict. If the 70 percent was sweet and the 80 percent was not sweet enough, but rather very bitter, then you're on your way, but not there yet. Continue following the diet more stringently and cut more sugar. If you try the 80 percent and it tastes a little sweet, while the 90 percent tastes bitter, you're about on track.

2. **Reduce your calories.** Even short-term calorie restriction can improve stem cell function. Try reducing your food intake by 20 percent for two weeks before you get your stem cells taken (making sure that you don't substitute sugar as above).

3. **Reduce your triglycerides.** Triglycerides (TRG) are the storage system in the blood for carbohydrates that go unused. This guideline goes hand in hand with the first two recommendations. TRG are also related to excess weight. One of our observations, which comes from years of culturing cells, is that stem cells grow poorly in patients with high TRG and in patients who are obese. Get your TRG measured and reduce your carbs and food intake to bring them

down to normal before you have your stem cells drawn. You may take a high-grade fish oil to help reduce your triglycerides. The recommended dose is at least four grams (4,000 milligrams) of EPA/DHA combined. The brand I recommend is Vital Nutrients. It comes in a liquid and is lemon flavored. Since it's highly purified, it doesn't have a fishy taste. It is also cost effective compared to taking capsules. Taking two teaspoons per day will give you five grams of EPA/DHA.

4. **As you are able, stay aerobically active and lift weights.** Research shows that more active older animals have better stem cells that create more bone, and weight lifters have better stem cells.[1] It also shows that exercise increases muscle stem cells. In our clinic, we have different activity level monikers: "PX90," "American Active," and "Couch Potato."

PX90 means eight to twelve hours a week of exercise hard enough that it would be tough to carry on a normal conversation during the activity. Examples include bike riding over mountains and at significant altitudes in 50–100-mile clips, running a trail for two hours with a 1,000-foot elevation gain, or scaling a 200-foot rock wall.

American Active denotes the usual health club exercise regimen. This generally includes cardiovascular work and using machines to lift weights for a high number of repetitions until a set number is reached.

Couch Potato means you don't do either of these. We want our patients (if feasible) to be somewhere between PX90 and American Active. This means that if you go to a gym, you should get a personal trainer to push you. If you lift weights with machines, do five to eight repetitions at a weight that will cause the muscle to fail, meaning you can't physically continue. If you run or bike, push yourself to go 20–30 percent faster or longer. If you're able, consider one of the popular cross fitness routines like Insanity or PX90.

What if your injuries preclude these workouts? Focus on things you can do. Consider water exercise. What if you're in poor shape with no hope of getting in better shape? Just up your activity levels to the best of your ability and concentrate on the other guidelines discussed in this list. Our goal is to extract the strongest stem cells we can, not necessarily to create elite athletes.

5. **Take supplements.** Refer to the nutritional guidelines in the prolotherapy and PRP sections earlier in this chapter, and also take vitamin D3 or get some outdoor time. Several studies show that D vitamins, D3 in particular, can help reduce stem cell aging, maintain their ability to turn into other needed cells, and make them healthier.[2]

6. **Take a stem cell supplement.** Either Stem X Cell or Ligagenix is fine. At this point, we don't have comparative data. Both can be found online.

7. **Take resveratrol for mitochondrial and telomere support.** Take 500 milligrams each day, mixed with 100 milligrams a day of ubiquinol. Several studies have shown that this will help MSCs differentiate and proliferate. In addition, this supplement may help control blood sugar.

8. **Low oxygen is better . . . sometimes.** You may consider a vacation to a high-altitude spot before your stem cell harvest. Even though you might not live at altitude, low oxygen levels consistent with high altitude help keep stem cells viable and growing. They differentiate better at normal oxygen

A NUMBER OF NUTRITIONAL SUPPLEMENTS MAY STRENGTHEN YOUR STEM CELLS OR CARTILAGE.

- **Curcumin:** Take 500 milligrams, three times per day
- **Quercetin:** Take 45 milligrams per day
- **Collagen Type 2:** Take 500 milligrams per day
- **Hyaluronic acid:** Take 50 milligrams per day
- **Manganese:** Take 10 milligrams per day
- **Vitamin C:** Take 1,000–2,000 milligrams per day
- **Zinc:** Take 50 milligrams per day
- **Stem X Cell and/or Ligagenix:** As directed
- **Arginine Plus:** Take 5,000 milligrams per day
- **Resveratrol:** Take 500 milligrams per day
- **Ubiquinol:** Take 100 milligrams per day
- **Glucosamine:** Take 1,500 milligrams per day
- **Chondroitin:** Take 1,200 milligrams per day
- **MSM:** Take 500 milligrams per day
- **Fish oil:** Take at least four grams per day
- **Vitamin D3:** Take 5,000 IU per day
- A high quality one-a-day vitamin with **B-complex and minerals**

levels. This may be why many elite athletes get benefit from sleeping in low-oxygen conditioning tents. There is a study showing that twenty hyperbaric oxygen (HBO) treatments can help the hematopoietic stem cells in bone marrow increase up to eight-fold prior to harvesting.

9. **Avoid prescription medications.** Based on our more than decade-long combined experience with stem cells at Regenexx, we have found that many prescription drugs hurt them. Time and time again, we have seen a patient's inabil-

ity to grow stem cells reverse when we take the patient off his medications. Getting off everything you can two to four weeks before the stem cell harvest is a good idea *as long as you clear it with the prescribing doctor.* We recommend staying off as many prescription medications as you can for six to twelve weeks after the reinjection of cells. The list of medications to avoid is based upon laboratory experiments performed with stem cells. Until further research is done with people taking these medications and having stem cell treatments, it is not certain these drugs will kill stem cells which have been injected into a patient. However, until the necessary research has been done, it is prudent to avoid as many prescription drugs as you can *with the approval of your prescribing physician.*

10. **Avoid all anti-inflammatory drugs.** These will prevent stem cells from growing and will depress healing. These include asthma medications such as Singulair, Advair, and Nasonex; as well as NSAIDs, including COX-2 inhibitors, such as Celebrex. Avoid them in all forms, including eye drops and skin creams.

11. **Avoid all steroids.** These will also prevent the stem cells from growing and will depress healing. This includes steroids in any form, including injections, oral, inhaled, topical, or drops. These should be avoided for three months prior to and following the procedure.

12. **Avoid quinalones and other antibiotics.** These can cause damage to tendons and ligaments, as well as possibly killing stem cells. Many people do not realize that some antibiotics include steroids.

13. **Avoid certain blood pressure medications, such as ACE inhibitors, ARBs, and AT-2 receptor antagonists.** Your doctor may elect to change your blood pressure medication to a stem cell-neutral medication, such as a calcium channel blocker.

14. **Avoid the statin class of drugs.** These medications, also called coenzyme reductase inhibitors and anti-lipid medication, have been shown to be detrimental to nerves, tendons, cartilage, and muscles. They also negatively affect the ability of stem cells to grow in culture.

15. **Avoid bisphosphonates for osteoporosis management.** Long-term use of these drugs is associated with jaw bone disease and spontaneous long bone fractures, as well as such short-term side effects as joint pain and soft tissue pain. They also negatively affect the ability of stem cells to grow in culture.

16. **Other medications that may interfere with stem cell treatments are:**
    - Some thyroid medications
    - Synthetic hormone supplements (Prempro)
    - Proton pump inhibitors (used to reduce gastric acid)
    - Avandia (for type-2 diabetes)
    - Interferon
    - Chemotherapy drugs
    - Propecia (for hair-loss)
    - Erythropoetin
    - Pepto-Bismol (because it contains salyciclates)
    - Artificial sweeteners

HELPING YOUR STEM CELLS GROW

The stem cell injection includes producing a micro-injury into the joint. As a result, expect the joint to be sore. This can be everything from minimally sore to extremely sore. If you have significant pain after your procedure, this should resolve within one to three weeks. If it does not resolve, contact your treating doctor.

1. **Prescription:** Take your narcotic pain medication as prescribed for more severe pain. Only use it as needed. Take it with food. Narcotic pain medicines can cause constipation, so increase fiber and fluids, and take a stool softener if needed. Acetaminophen is okay for mild pain. For bone-healing conditions, like AVN and non-union fractures, we will prescribe Calcitonin Nasal Spray. Spray one time each day.

2. **Blood flow.** Infrared light therapy is recommended to help maintain the life of the stem cells during their implantation phase. Infrared heating pads can be purchased online. The treatment protocol is thirty minutes twice a day for six weeks after the stem cells are implanted.

3. **Supplements:** Recommended are those on the list below.
   - **Collagen type 2:** Take 500 milligrams per day
   - **Hyaluronic acid:** Take 50 milligrams per day
   - **Manganese:** Take 10 milligrams per day
   - **Vitamin C:** Take 1,000–2,000 milligrams per day
   - **Zinc:** Take 50 milligrams per day
   - **Stem X Cell or Ligagenix:** As directed
   - **Arginine Plus:** Take 5,000 milligrams per day
   - **Resveratrol:** Take 500 milligrams per day
   - **Ubiquinol:** Take 100 milligrams per day
   - **Glucosamine:** Take 1,500 milligrams per day
   - **Chondroitin:** Take 1,200 milligrams per day

- **MSM:** Take 500 milligrams per day
- **Fish oil:** Take 2 grams per day
- **Vitamin D3:** Take 5,000 IU per day
- A high quality one-a-day multivitamin with **B-complex and minerals**

4. **Avoid:** Do not take the following supplements for at least six weeks after the stem cells are injected. These supplements at higher doses may have a negative anti-inflammatory effect on the treatment area.
   - **Curcumin**
   - **Quercetin**
   - Reduce your **fish oil** to only 2 grams a day

5. **Follow the same recommendations for prescription medications as you did prior to your stem cell treatment.**
6. **Alcohol and marijuana:** Alcohol can have a profound negative effect on stem cell function, so this should be avoided for six to twelve weeks after your stem cell treatment. A glass of wine with dinner is all right, but more than this should be avoided. Cannaboids, such as marijuana, can promote bone formation over cartilage when working on cartilage damage in joints. This is not what we want to happen in this case, so it should be avoided.
7. **Diet:** Continue low-carbohydrate diet for six to twelve more weeks to suppress formation of triglycerides, as these can interfere with stem cell survival.

ACTIVITY AFTER A STEM CELL TREATMENT

The goal of the treatment is to allow the stem cells to attach to areas of damage and then protect them while they differentiate into cartilage. For this reason, you'll be asked to keep the joint as still as possible for thirty to sixty minutes after the procedure. Do not take a bath for three days, but a shower twelve hours after the procedure is fine.

1. For the first three days after treatment, you should limit activity on the joint. This may be easy to do if you have post-operative soreness, as you may have a natural limp or "antalgic" gait (your body does this to reduce pressure on the area to allow healing). If you don't have this, then taking weight off this area as you walk by using crutches or a cane is a good idea the first two days. Avoid all contact sports, as well as jogging, running, or sports that involve impact on that joint.

2. From the fourth through fourteenth days after treatment, you can start to walk normally for no more than thirty to sixty minutes per day. Avoid all contact sports, as well as jogging, running, or sports that involve impact on that joint. Bike riding is fine, as are stationary bike, swimming and, after the tenth day, elliptical machines.

3. From the third through sixth weeks after treatment, continue to avoid all contact sports, as well as jogging, running, or sports that involve impact on that joint. You can walk as much as you like on the joint now.

4. Six weeks after treatment, start reintegrating all desired activities into your regimen, adding back 20 percent per week. For example, if you were used to running twenty miles a week, start at four miles a week and then add an-

other four miles per week, and so on. The stem cell injection includes producing a micro-injury into the joint. As a result expect the joint to be sore. This can be everything from minimally sore to very sore.

UNLOADER BRACES AFTER A STEM CELL PROCEDURE

If you have a significant loss of cartilage and meniscus damage in one compartment of the knee, or what may be an unstable meniscus tear, our center uses an unloader brace after the stem cells are transplanted into that area. The purpose is to reduce forces on these cells while still allowing for weight-bearing activity and cyclic loading (the type of intermittent pressure that comes from walking). This will help the cells differentiate into cartilage or help repair a torn meniscus. These braces can be expensive. Here's what you should know.

1. These braces come in a left and right model.
2. These braces come in either a medial or lateral compartment unloader. This means they can either take pressure off the inner (medial) or outer (lateral) side of the knee joint. For example, if you lost the cartilage on the inside of your right knee, you are looking for a right medial unloader brace.
3. Your unloader brace needs to be adjustable. Most models are. Your brace fitter will teach you how to adjust your brace. Ideally, we want the brace adjusted to a maximum amount you can tolerate to keep the joint open short of causing pain from the excessive pressure on your skin. This is important because too much pressure can irritate or cause skin break down. Over the six weeks of wear, it is recommended to back off the adjustment a little each week. However, if you

find a spot where the brace makes the knee feel better, keep it there during the six-week healing period. Some patients with a severe angle deformity will find the brace will help them long term, which is just fine.

4. Size matters. Braces come in different lengths, meaning how long they extend up and down your leg, as well as different circumferences, meaning how snugly they fit around your leg.

5. I recommend an off-the-shelf unloader for those who will only need the brace for six weeks. It will be billed through your insurance if you have durable medical equipment coverage. Your doctor's staff will help determine how much out-of-pocket expense you will incur if you are required to pay a deductible or a co-payment. If you need a long-term brace, the doctor will order a permanent semi-custom or custom brace that will last much longer.

6. I recommend a post-operative shoulder brace for full-thickness rotator cuff repairs and a Richie brace or a walking boot for cartilage stem cell repair in ankles.

YOUR EXPERIENCE MAY VARY

Some physicians may do things differently than I have described.

1. Some physicians use lasers or electromagnetic treatments as adjuncts to their RIT work. I await more scientific evidence before I add these after treatments for my RIT patients.

2. While some physicians do not use lidocaine, new research has shown that if the dosage is low, there doesn't seem to be a negative effect from the use of this numbing agent even if it comes into direct contact with the area into which the stem cells are being injected. Lidocaine and ropivacaine in

low dose also makes treatments a lot more comfortable and tolerable for the patient.

CONTRAINDICATIONS FOR RIT

1. Regenerative injection therapy cannot be used to treat every patient. For example: If you have an underlying disease that already compromises your immune system—from a cold virus to uncontrolled HIV, hepatitis, cancer, or Lyme disease—it is going to be more difficult for you to heal well. Uncontrolled or poorly controlled diabetes could interfere with these treatments. When the system is already stressed from one imbalance, it cannot be as effective in dealing with another.

2. If you have a history of any allergies—especially to lidocaine, steroids, latex, cod fish, or corn syrup, all of which may be factors in the treatments offered to you—you may not be a candidate for RIT. Discuss your specific needs with your doctor.

3. If you are taking antibiotics, are being treated for an infection, or are feeling ill, postpone your treatment until after you are well.

4. If you cannot cease medications that could interfere with the treatment, you may not be a candidate for RIT. We know that NSAIDs, cortisone, and other anti-inflammatory drugs and blood thinners do interfere. We suspect that some antibiotics and cholesterol-lowering drugs (statins) also do. Also being studied, particularly for their interaction with ASCI, are bisphosphonates (osteoporosis drugs), angiotensin-converting-enzyme (ACE) inhibitors, and angiotensin II receptor blockers (ARB). Blood thinners pres-

ent a bleeding risk that, in certain circumstances, could make treatments dangerous for patients to undergo.

INDICATIONS THAT SOMETHING IS WRONG

Contact your doctor's office or go to the emergency room if you experience any of the following signs or symptoms after an RIT treatment.

1. An allergic reaction such as shortness of breath, hives, or itching. Mild itching around the injection site for several days after the treatment is normal and can be controlled with any low-dose, over-the-counter steroid cream or diphenhydramine.
2. Any signs of infection, such as redness, warmth, drainage, severe swelling, a red line radiating toward the trunk of your body, or a fever.
3. A hyper-inflammatory response marked by increasing pain and discomfort, particularly if it lasts longer than five days.
4. Any headaches, particularly after spine injections, and especially if they worsen after you stand and improve when you lie down.

CHAPTER FOURTEEN
WHY DO I HAVE TO PAY OUT OF POCKET?

One of the questions patients most often ask me is, "Why won't my insurance pay for these treatments?" I answer that most insurance companies, at this time, consider regenerative injection therapies to be experimental and not yet within the mainstream standard of care. As I have explained in this book, more than one million people in this country have been treated with these methods. Prolotherapy has been used since the 1930s, giving it an over eighty-year track record. A similar treatment technique, sclerotherapy, is an accepted treatment for dealing with spider veins, varicose veins, and hemorrhoids. Platelet-rich plasma has been used since the 1970s and is an accepted treatment for a number of illnesses, including severe burns. Bone marrow, for its rich supply of stem cells, is regularly transplanted for some forms of cancer and blood disease. There are other countries in the world where some of the RIT treatments are more commonly used and accepted as a standard of care.

All of the foregoing would demonstrate that these older forms of RIT are "experimental" with an enormous amount of real-life, positive proof. Still, U.S. insurance companies today are not willing to extend coverage to musculoskeletal uses for these treatments. Ironically, if they did, they could potentially save billions of dollars they now pay for surgery and medications that might prove unnecessary if RIT were more available.

In the United States, it costs in the neighborhood of $800 million dollars in testing and marketing, and takes about twelve years, to get a new drug approved by the Food and Drug Administration (FDA) and then covered by insurance and marketed to the general public.[1] Because regenerative injection techniques uti-

---

It costs in the neighborhood of $800 million dollars in testing and marketing, and takes about twelve years, to get a new drug approved by the FDA.

---

lize common, easily accessible solutions, like dextrose, lidocaine, autologous blood, and stem cells, there is no financial incentive for a pharmaceutical company to invest in testing and research. Centrifuges used for PRP and ASCI are already manufactured and in use. There is no incentive for a medical equipment company to make that investment. Consequently, it is difficult for RIT researchers to find the funding they need to conduct the studies that would make this treatment acceptable to insurers.

According to evidence-based medicine rules, a new treatment becomes accepted as the standard of care when two or more high-level research studies (called Level Ia studies) have positive outcomes. This is construed to show that the intended results of the treatment works more effectively than a control treatment. Without such large, controlled studies showing beyond a shadow of a doubt that RIT works better than a placebo, it is unlikely to be covered. Although there have been about one hundred research projects published on prolotherapy in the past, most of them have been Level II to Level IV studies. Few have been Level I studies, which means they were sizable, randomized, and controlled trials of the quality that could move RIT toward widespread acceptance.[2]

At the time of writing, there are a number of Level I studies in their final stages or working their way towards publication. These studies concern prolotherapy's effect on knee arthritis, growth plate injuries in children, and tennis elbow. When they are all published, there will be more than two Level I studies showing the efficacy of RIT treatment.

The National Institute of Health (NIH) funded a five-year knee arthritis study of over 150 people, conducted by Jeffrey Patterson, D.O., and David Rabago, M.D., from the University of Wisconsin. Patterson and Rabago have designed the study and written up articles concerning it. The first of their articles was published very recently.[3] The rest were pending publication at the time I wrote this book. An NIH study can be a decisive factor in a treatment's acceptance. In the Level I study of one hundred randomized patients, fifty were getting prolotherapy and fifty were getting saline injections. However, in the randomized control trial, the prolotherapy-treated patients had better pain control and function, and less stiffness than the patients in the control group. In the concomitant Level II study, there were fifty non-randomized patients who had a pre-existing bias in favor of prolotherapy. For these patients, possible variables were taken into account, but it was not considered Level I research, given the preexisting bias of the patients and their foreknowledge of their treatment. Consequently, their results could be considered to be tainted by the possibility of an undocumented placebo effect.

An article published by Dean Reeves, M.D., and Gaston Topol, M.D., in *Pediatrics* in 2011 was based upon a Level I study of young athletes suffering from a condition called Osgood-Schlatter disease,[4] which is an irritation of the growth center where the patella tendon attaches to the upper shin bone. I wrote about this condition in Chapter Twelve, recounting the story of Lucille, who had suffered from the disease as a child. In this study, entitled "Hyperosmolar Dextrose Injections for Recalcitrant Osgood-Schlatter Disease," it was concluded that treatment with prolotherapy produced a superior symptom reduction in adolescents. It was also concluded that the treatment was safe and well tolerated, and resulted in more rapid and frequent return to play without pain from symptoms.

Another Level I study by Scarpone and Rabago was reported in the *Clinical Journal of Sports Medicine* in 2008.[5] In this study, adults with tennis elbow received either prolotherapy or saline injections. The study concluded that prolotherapy effectively decreased elbow pain and improved strength testing compared to the control group. It was also well-tolerated.

Both of these studies were considered to be excellent pilot studies, well-designed with good statistics. However, there were insufficient participants to enable the studies to qualify as Level Ia studies.

Reeves and Topol are also the lead researchers on several studies that are being performed in Argentina. In that country, there is less bias among the medical community against prolotherapy. However, studies done there and in other countries are sometimes discounted in America. Reeves and Topol's study is looking at the effect of prolotherapy on advanced osteoarthritis of the knee and hip. They have found that after a year of treatment with prolotherapy, areas of joints which had been completely devoid of cartilage at the beginning of the study showed some hyaline cartilage growth.[6] I will discuss their study in detail in Chapter Fifteen.

Will RIT remain outside mainstream U.S. medicine's "standard of care," only available to patients from physicians who, like me, seek to treat their patients with any treatment that has a reasonable research record, is safe and works on real people? I don't

---

If enough people learn about RIT and want it to be available, they can make their desire known to their physicians, governmental representatives, employers, friends, and relatives.

---

think so. I believe RIT will eventually be considered part of the accepted standard of care for many musculoskeletal conditions. It's just a matter of time. With doctors like Rabago, Scarpone, Patterson, and Reeves committed to doing the hard work of significant research, we are very close to widespread acceptance of these treatment methods.

There are several ways in which this can happen. The first one is part of the reason I have written this book. If enough people learn about RIT and want it to be available as a treatment, they can make their desire known to their physicians, to their governmental representatives, to their employers, and to their friends and relatives. Having learned about the possibilities of RIT, I trust you will begin to question why it is not practiced by more physicians or covered by insurance.

It is my opinion, and the opinion of others, like Dean Reeves, M.D., that the second method of acceptance will come when lawyers begin to question doctors in personal injury or malpractice suits about why they did not treat a patient with RIT. This is where the Level I studies come in: Two such studies provide sufficient scientific evidence for a treatment to no longer be considered experimental. Consequently, it becomes part of the accepted standard of care, and allows lawyers the opportunity to contend that ignoring RIT as an acceptable treatment option could be considered negligent. An expert witness will testify that he would have treated a patient's injuries with prolotherapy, which is the standard of care for x, y, or z.

Let's take the example of a hypothetical tennis elbow injury that had a poor outcome. The lawyer could make the argument that since this patient had failed conventional standard of care treatments, he should have been offered a course of RIT before going to surgery. Instead, he underwent a surgery that rendered him permanently disabled. The lawyer would have his expert witness testify there is randomized, controlled, Level I evidence showing that RIT might have helped this patient so he could have avoided surgery. If the defendant in that case ended up being found liable because he didn't refer the patient for prolotherapy, that would establish a legal precedent. Eventually, such a precedent would spread throughout the country. If doctors start losing cases for not using or recommending RIT, many more doctors would advocate for it being an accepted and reimbursable method of treatment.

The political arena provides the third way in which RIT could be accepted. Just as there are representatives who are pro-stem cell research, there are pro-prolotherapy representatives as well. I know one of them personally. Apparently, this congressman and his brother were athletes in their youth. When they were injured, the doctor they saw in Chicago helped them dramatically with injections. Being young, they didn't really think much about the treatment. It later came up when the congressman's wife was injured and searching for a treatment for her injury. The congressman learned that the doctor he and his brother had seen was Gustav Anders Hemwall, M.D., the founder of the Hackett-Hemwall Foundation. The congressman contacted me, since he was interested in drafting legislation in favor of prolotherapy being an accepted treatment. At that time, there was not enough Level I evidence to support passage of such legislation. Now, there is. However, the people reading and interpreting the studies for the interested members of Congress would be doctors, most likely orthopedic surgeons, not interventional orthopedic doctors or integrative orthopedic medicine doctors. I trust, however, that the research would speak for itself.

Political intervention on a state level may also help RIT become a more widely accepted treatment. An interesting recent example comes from Governor Rick Perry of Texas, who had his spinal problem successfully treated with autologous stem cells in 2011.[7] He has since attempted to make Texas a state that is friendly to all forms of stem cell research and treatment.[8] However, he has encountered problems with the FDA, which is attempting to stop research in the state that does not correspond with its minimal manipulation ruling and other rulings.

In my opinion, it is inevitable that RIT will, in one of the ways discussed in this chapter, become a well-established treatment technique. When RIT is considered part of the accepted standard of care for musculoskeletal conditions, then you will no longer need to pay for it out of your own pocket.

CHAPTER FIFTEEN
WHAT EVERY DOCTOR SHOULD KNOW ABOUT RIT

This chapter should be read by every physician who treats patients suffering from musculoskeletal injuries or pain. Whether you have considered utilizing or referring patients for interventional orthopedics, integrative orthopedic medicine, or regenerative injection therapy, you will find something here that will make you a better doctor. I strongly recommend this chapter to all ancillary health care practitioners who work in this field. I anticipate that many medically responsible patients will also find this chapter highly educational.

Knowing firsthand how busy health care practitioners are today, in this chapter I am going to give you shortcuts to understand and to explain the new, regenerative-healing paradigm and RIT to your patients. I will discuss the medical, scientific, political, and financial issues surrounding the new paradigm, and will address questions you may still have. I started my journey to this paradigm with many questions myself. After a decade of studying and empirically using these methods, I have answered many of these questions. I have also been able to better understand what needs to be done in the medical and research communities to obtain some of the other answers. I trust this chapter will dispel your doubts and engage your interest enough to encourage you to consider giving the new paradigm of musculoskeletal healing the respect it is due. Perhaps it will even encourage some physicians and other health-care professionals to obtain thorough and proper training in some aspects of this new healing paradigm.

I am presenting this chapter as a list of frequently asked questions to enable you to find the information you need easily and quickly. For continuing and updated information, follow my website: www.Regen4Life.com.

QUESTIONS CONCERNING THE NEW PARADIGM

What is the new healing paradigm?
The new paradigm is a methodology rooted in the belief that the body has the ability to heal itself, either naturally or by being given a push in the right direction. This push can come from manipulation, physical therapy, correct use of medication, or regenerative injection treatments.

How does it differ from how doctors treat orthopedic patients now?
Conceptually, the new paradigm looks at a bigger picture, with an eye to making an accurate diagnosis, developing a comprehensive treatment plan that works, and preventing further injury. Practically, this means that new-paradigm practitioners are always considering the kinetic chain, reflex inhibition, postural decompensation, dynamic stabilization failure, and concomitant medical issues affecting a patient's musculoskeletal health. Practitioners use old, but underutilized orthopedic methods, integrative medical solutions, and interventional orthopedics. including regenerative injection treatments.

What is the field of interventional orthopedics?

Interventional orthopedics uses minimally invasive proce-dures to treat and hopefully cure orthopedic conditions that until now, would have been treated with arthroscopic or open surgi-cal techniques. It places an emphasis on regenerative injection treatments where appropriate. Along with other physicians, I am working to make interventional orthopedics a non-surgical sub-specialty.

Is it different from integrative orthopedic medicine?

Yes, it is. Integrative orthopedic medicine employs a holistic approach to a patient with an orthopedic condition. Beyond the traditional treatments used in orthopedics, sports medicine or physiatry, doctors who practice this specialty also consider the medical aspects of the patient's orthopedic condition. This would include hormone imbalance, nutrition, and vitamin supplemen-tation. The methodology of integrative orthopedic medicine is to use all reasonable ancillary approaches to help the patient's orthopedic condition to heal. This is a medical approach to or-thopedic injuries, rather than a surgical one.

Beyond the obvious, what happens when a patient is injured?

Old-paradigm musculoskeletal medicine does not always suf-ficiently emphasize the kinetic chain. Any injury can affect this whole chain, later contributing to reflex inhibition, dynamic sta-bilization failure, and postural decompensation. Because of the interlocking nature of the kinetic chain, something as simple as a sprained ankle, insufficiently treated, can set the stage for pre-mature disability and degenerative arthritis.

An injury, particularly if it becomes chronic, can also cause major changes in a patient's hormone balance, thus affecting mood, energy level, appetite, sleep, and the capacity to heal.

How are you using ultrasound?

I use ultrasound as a diagnostic tool. An ultrasound machine, when properly used, is capable of giving better spatial resolution hence a much clearer picture of superficial structure problems than an MRI. Diagnostic ultrasound is capable of magnifying the area in question several times over, while an MRI usually shrinks the image relative to the structure of interest.

I also use ultrasound for guiding injections accurately into pathologic tissue. Injecting a small amount of anesthetic into the tissue in question during such a procedure might also identify occult tears. The hydrostatic pressure of the injected fluid can open a tear that could otherwise remain invisible to either an ultrasound or an MRI.

What do you mean by "underused methods" of treating patients?

There are many labor-intensive methods of treating injuries that have been set aside in favor of medications and surgical interventions, which require less time. Some of the underused methods are as simple as prescribing orthotics or testing a patient's gait. Others are as complex as manipulating a patient using osteopathic, chiropractic, or myofascial release technique. A good new-paradigm practitioner strives to be connected to a network of excellent practitioners of ancillary therapies, to which he can refer patients.

QUESTIONS CONCERNING YOUR DOUBTS

What evidence is there that there's any validity to what you are doing?

I can attest to the benefits of RIT from my own experiences as a patient, as outlined in Chapter Two, "My Journey to Regenerative Healing." Additionally, I have had the experience of treating more than ten thousand patients and seeing the positive results of these treatments.

Apart from this anecdotal evidence, I get my data from the literature, and from attending relevant conferences and courses. Is the data I have gathered flawed? Of course, but only as much as any other orthopedic literature is. Ideally we will review and change our practice of medicine when high quality Level I studies are introduced and vetted by our medical community. However, until then we have to make the best treatment decisions we can for our patients. Cutting-edge doctors still rely on case reports and case series as a way to get a first look at a new treatment or procedural technique. When the standard of care has failed our patients for a chance for a cure, then we will use all available evidence and experience to try to successfully treat our patients. Some call this courageous and others call it irresponsible.

As a resident and sports medicine fellow, I learned how to read the data and the literature surrounding an experiment. As a fellowship director, I taught others how to do the same. I have also done research on both tennis elbow and hamstring injuries. Both of these were five-year projects. One was published, and the other was presented at national conferences. Currently, I am journal editor for *Clinical Journal of Sports Medicine, Global Advances in Health and Medicine, Annals of Family Medicine, Physical*

Medicine and Rehabilitation Journal, and *The American Journal of Sports Medicine.* Through all of this, I have learned to evaluate research and watch for irrational leaps of faith. Remember, everything has a bias. I know how to watch for someone's pre-existing bias against or for a treatment, which can influence the study design and/or his summary of an article or research project.

Many doctors, especially those in academics or research, believe that evidence-based medicine is the only way to proceed. However, there can be fatal flaws in evidence-based medicine's analysis of orthopedic research. In addition, to design a study that is doable and affordable, often what happens in the trenches of our medical practices has to be watered down so far that the treatment being studied no longer resembles real-life practice. To illustrate this, I will evaluate here three articles about prolotherapy and PRP, that have been used to discredit these methods. I use these articles to give examples of how fatal flaws can lead to inaccurate conclusions.

1. Michael J. Yelland, et al., "Prolotherapy Injections, Saline Injections, and Exercises for Chronic, Low-Back Pain: A Randomized Trial," *Spine,* 2004.

This is one of the landmark studies that led Medicare, once again, to refuse to approve prolotherapy as a reimbursable treatment. It was interpreted as a negative-outcome study for the effect of prolotherapy on low back pain.

There were 110 patients enrolled in the study. They all had low back pain for an average of fourteen years. The study group patients received injections of 20-percent dextrose with 0.2-percent lidocaine. The patients in the control got injections of normal saline with 0.2-percent lidocaine. Both groups received injections into the lumbosacral spine ligament system. The groups were randomized to receive either exercise or normal activity over six months. They were injected every two weeks and evaluated at twelve and twenty-four months. One hundred and nine patients completed a survey at six months, 106 at twelve months, and eighty-eight at two years. The outcome reported that most patients experienced a significant decrease of pain and disability. However, there was no significant difference between groups. Adverse effects included low back pain and stiffness, an increase in leg pain, nausea, spinal headaches, and thoracic pain. These were widespread among participants and classified as short-term adverse events, since most lasted fewer than five days.

The most likely reason there was no difference between treatment groups was due to the study design. Injecting the atypical large amount of fluid used (three cubic centimeters) into each ligament, whether saline or dextrose, would likely cause a tissue change. Therefore a large-volume saline injection is not a good control to use in prolotherapy studies.

A study by Klein had a similar design, but used a small amount of saline vs. dextrose injected into the ligaments of the lower back.[1, 2] This study saw a significant difference between groups. In Yellend's study, both groups got significantly better than baseline: In fact, they got the same or more relief than is customarily seen in spinal surgery studies. This is further support for the fact that a large-volume saline injection is not a good control. Rather, it is an active treatment when it performs as well as other treatment solutions. Finally, more evidence that saline is not a good control is the fact that the control group in Yelland's study experienced the same side effects as the experimental group did: the classic increase in pain and stiffness for several days after the treatment.

This study needs to be reproduced and redesigned using up-to-date standard, U.S. prolotherapy treatment protocols which new-paradigm physicians are trained to perform. In these, the amount of dextrose injected into each target site is three to six times less than the amount used in the Yelland study. Based on our current prolotherapy experience, the amount of adverse events Yelland's study reported would indicate the amount of solution injected caused a much higher incidence of side effects, albeit temporary ones, than we are accustomed to seeing in our practices.

2. Robert J. De Vos, et al. "Platelet-rich Plasma Injection for Chronic Achilles Tendinopathy," *Journal of the American Medical Association*, 2010.

This was a PRP study of treatments for chronic Achilles tendon disease. It was a randomized study, where fifty-four patients received either PRP or saline injections into the diseased Achilles tendon using ultrasound guidance. Both groups were also given an eccentric exercise program. Both groups had significant improvement in both pain and function.

There were several problems with this study. Number one, the exercise given to both groups is the only evidence-based treatment shown to work for chronic Achilles tendon disease. The addition of the injection therapy did not make a statistical increase in the amount of improvement in each group.

The issue that one has to consider in studying the effectiveness of healing Achilles tendinopathy with a combination of evidence-based protocol and an additional treatment is that the design of the experiment, where the study was conducted with so few patients, would make it difficult to ascertain whether the additional treatment enhanced healing. Constructing a study this way would be like doing a strep throat study in which both groups received penicillin. However, the experimental group also received gummy bears, whereas the control group received a sugar pill. From this study design, the researchers could conclude that gummy bears do not help cure strep throat. In a similar fashion, the doctors performing this study concluded that PRP did not produce a significantly greater healing effect than saline.

Number two, in the injection part of the study the patients were only treated one time, and the number of needle passes into the diseased area was arbitrarily set at five per injection area, with fifteen injections overall, at four ccs total volume of solution. The problem with this is that no expert in the field of sports medicine who performs PRP for Achilles tendon cases would offer only a single treatment: the average number of treatments to cure—or at least to bring a patient through s post-injection, eccentric training exercise program—is three to four, not one. The other issue is that placing 0.3 ccs of PRP in fifteen areas on a diseased tendon is not as comprehensive a treatment as sports medicine-trained PRP experts would follow in their usual clinical practices. We usually inject up to double this amount in a heavily diseased Achilles tendon. The amount of needling could be triple the amount done in the study. The idea is to penetrate the tendon with twenty-five to one hundred needle passes, depending on the state of the disease, until the needle passes smoothly through the diseased tendon. The PRP is then injected into the needled area.

The final problem of this study was that it used a lab-created, single-centrifugation PRP product. My associates at Regenexx have discovered this type of PRP yields only a one- to two-times baseline platelet concentration. This is not platelet-rich plasma. Rather, it is platelet-poor plasma. In my experience, this low of a platelet concentration greatly lessens a patient's ability to heal.

3. Scott A. Rodeo, et al., "Platelet-rich Plasma in Rotator Cuff Repair," *Techniques in Orthopedics,* 2007.

The main problem with this study, which used PRP to treat patients who were having rotator cuff surgical repair, is similar to one of the problems with the De Vos study: The researchers used the Cascade system, which only concentrates the platelets to one to two times baseline concentration. This might be adequate for minor conditions, but is not a platelet-rich plasma treatment. The bottom line is that Cascade and Arthrex are single-spin centrifuge systems that only achieve limited platelet concentration. Scott Rodeo has demonstrated in other studies that he is knowledgeable about different PRP products and manufacturing techniques, so why did he choose a system he was likely to know was only capable of producing an inferior healing effect?

One of the criticisms the research community as a whole holds against PRP is that there haven't been enough animal studies to proceed to human ones. To experiment on one hundred dogs is a $1 million-dollar study, which is the same amount it costs for a one-year orthopedic study with one hundred people. It can take twenty years to progress from animal studies to human practice. It is only after producing a couple of years' worth of papers on animal studies on a technique to prove that it isn't harmful, that you move to human studies. All those studies are expensive and labor intensive. Normally after proceeding through the basic science and bench research with animals, you then progress through phases I—IV in human trials.

In the 1980s, doctors used PRP in burn studies and dental research because there was nothing else to offer that might work. Rodeo could be right that PRP is not ready for orthopedic use in humans because we don't have sufficient research at this time. However, it is being used on orthopedic problems for which we really don't have an effective standard of care treatment at this time, much as it was earlier for seemingly unsolvable burn and jaw reconstruction disease states. Given the good PRP has apparently done, it should be tested fairly and not used in a study that damns it by design.

Why aren't there more studies about these methods?

A Level I blinded, randomized control trial costs about $1 million dollars per year to study one hundred people at the university setting. A Level I study attempts to remove the element of bias from a group of patients receiving an experimental treatment and compares the results against a control group. Neither the doctors providing the treatment nor the patients receiving it know who got the experimental or the control treatment. If you have over one hundred patients in an orthopedic study, this is considered to be a large study.

In other fields of medicine, a large study would follow at least 200 patients, or many more, for a fraction of the cost. A Level II study is an uncontrolled or single-blinded study, meaning that either the patient or doctor may know the patient is receiving the experimental agent being studied. A Level III study is a case series where the cases are usually analyzed after the treatment has been performed. A Level IV study consists of evidence provided by experts' opinions and is weighted about the same as anecdotal evidence.

Are there any Level I studies showing these RIT methods work?

A study funded by the National Institutes of Health (NIH) and the National Center for Complementary and Alternative Medicine was recently completed at the University of Wisconsin,[3] led by David Rabago, M.D., who has dedicated his research career to studying prolotherapy. He was a teacher before he became a physician, and he chose to work in the university setting to enable him to do the most research. There is a lot of evidence today about prolotherapy because of people like Drs. Rabago, Patterson, Scarpone, and Reeves, who have been conducting high-quality RIT research constantly for the past decade. The NIH study was a five-year, $5 million-dollar project to study the effect of prolotherapy on osteoarthritis of the knee. The study consisted of a randomized, controlled trial, as well as an unblinded, prospective case-controlled series. In the randomized, controlled trial, some patients received dextrose; others, saline; the rest, exercise alone.

Although the results have not yet been published, there was a poster presentation of this study at the Osteoarthritis Research Society International (OARSI) World Congress on Osteoarthritis in 2011.[4] The study concluded that prolotherapy "resulted in safe, significant, sustained improvement of pain, function, and stiffness scores, compared to blinded saline injections and at-home exercises in knee osteoarthritis . . . Satisfaction with prolotherapy was high, and there were no adverse events."[5]

This was also the result of the case-controlled series. The first installment of the results of the latter series was published in the April 2012 issue of *The Journal of Alternative and Complementary Medicine*. When the randomized, controlled trial results are published, it is expected that they will be classified as a Level Ia study.

There are also two excellent Level Ib studies that have been published. The first, entitled "Hyperosmolar Dextrose Injections for Recalcitrant Osgood-Schlatter Disease," appeared in November 2011 in *Pediatrics*.[6] This study concluded that treatment with prolotherapy produced superior symptom reduction in adolescents suffering from an irritation of the growth center where the patella tendon attaches to the upper shin bone (Osgood-Schlatter disease). The study also concluded the treatment was safe, well tolerated, and achieved a more rapid return to play without pain from activity.

The other study, entitled "The Efficacy of Prolotherapy for Lateral Epicondylitis: A Pilot Study," was reported by Michael Scarpone, D.O., in *The Clinical Journal of Sports Medicine* in 2008.[7] In this study, adults with tennis elbow received either prolotherapy or saline injections. The study concluded that the prolotherapy effectively decreased elbow pain, improved strength testing, and was well tolerated. David Rabago, M.D., is currently leading a pilot study evaluating thirty patients with tennis elbow who have not responded to conventional treatment.[8] In this randomized, controlled trial, he is using a disease-specific, validated outcome measure to determine whether prolotherapy is effective.

Both the Osgood-Schlatter and the tennis elbow studies are considered to be excellent pilots, well designed and with good statistics. However, there were insufficient participants in any of these studies to enable them to qualify for Level Ia status.

As noted in Chapter Fourteen, Drs. Dean Reeves and Gaston Topol presented their interim findings from their prolotherapy studies in Argentina at a symposium in 2012. Their group has been studying the effects of prolotherapy on advanced osteoarthritis of both the knee and hip.[9] Specifically, they wanted to determine whether prolotherapy would have any effect on regenerating hyaline cartilage. First, they performed arthroscopic surgery on the knees and hips to observe the amount of cartilage loss and put methylene blue stain inside the patients' joints. This stain is only absorbed by good hyaline cartilage. Their images showed large areas that were bright white from lack of cartilage, and areas with cartilage that absorbed the dye that were deep blue. Second, during the surgery researchers used arthroscopic cameras to view and photograph the extent of cartilage damage before the study started. Third, they performed biopsies on the arthritic areas to assess the quality of the existing cartilage.

Following this initial work, the researchers administered a prolotherapy injection into the joint every other month for a year. At the end of the study, they repeated the initial arthroscopic surgery protocols listed above. They observed that in a significant number of patients, joints which had been completely devoid of cartilage at the beginning of the study showed significant hyaline-like cartilage growth. In many of these patients, biopsies showed normal cartilage–bone interface. This is exciting work. Researchers in the stem cell field are developing very expensive research protocols to try to achieve the same goal that this study seems to already show: simple dextrose prolotherapy has the power to regenerate cartilage in advanced arthritis. Understand, these are preliminary results and the full story on the outcome of this study is still a couple of years away.

Why aren't there more Level I research projects on these methods?
As I mentioned earlier, a Level I, randomized, controlled trial in the field of orthopedics costs about $1 million dollars per year to study one hundred people in the university setting. Because

the medications and medical equipment used for RIT already exists, no pharmaceutical or medical equipment company stands to recoup expenses from making such an investment. That leaves private clinics and governmental or academic institutions as the potential sources of funding. Since the downturn in the economy, the potential resources for our government to fund RIT research have all but dried up. That leaves private clinics that cannot afford to design and fund a high-quality study.

The only way the type of studies that need to be published can be developed and run is going to be through private funding. I propose that those of us interested in new-paradigm healing, as a group, have the power to help fund this research privately with our own donations. This is not a new concept, and it is one that has worked before. In the near future, I will develop a non-profit research fund where doctors, patients, friends, and families can donate money to fund a research trust. From this trust, doctors such as Rabago, Scarpone, Reeves, Centeno, and I will be able to apply for grants to fund high-quality RIT research. Such research can begin to prove definitively how well RIT stacks up against conventional treatments.

Is research being done in other parts of the world?

In addition to the work being done in Argentina, there is also an ongoing tennis elbow study being conducted in Australia.

In Korea, Young Uck Kim, M.D., is a physician who runs an orthopedic hospital. One floor of his hospital is dedicated to offering prolotherapy. Dr. Kim has given presentations on several case reports and case series that he has treated.[10]

There is a variety of work being done in many parts of Europe. In Germany, a form of PRP that does not fall under the FDA's minimal manipulation rule is being practiced, and it is popular with elite athletes from around the world. It is purported that this treatment, called Orthokine, can allow a patient with a horribly arthritic knee to run as though he has no injury. The procedure takes whole blood and incubates the blood for a time with glass beads. This causes the platelets to secrete certain anti-inflammatory growth factors and reduce Interleukin 1, a pro-inflammatory growth factor, to levels that can help get a badly arthritic joint under good pain control for many months.[11] Los Angeles Lakers shooting guard Kobe Bryant swears by the treatment and credits its effect for his renewed ability to play at a competitive level.[12] Doctors in Italy, Greece, Turkey, China, Asia, Israel, South America, and South Africa are also researching RIT and reporting their findings at international conferences.

Because of the international trips made by the Hackett-Hemwall Foundation (HHF) and the American Academy of Osteopathy (AAO), doctors have been trained in RIT in Canada, Honduras, the Philippines, South Africa, Mexico, Peru, Egypt, Hong Kong, South Korea, Italy, and mainland China.

Can RIT continue to be ignored by the mainstream for much longer?

No, it is on the verge of being accepted by mainstream medicine in the very near future. New York University has just decided to open a clinic that will feature prolotherapy, and one of the doctors there called me for advice about how to set things up.

One of the organizations with which I am associated, the American Association of Orthopaedic Medicine (AAOM), was recently contacted by Health Canada to explore the possibility of utilizing prolotherapy as a mainstream standard of care for musculoskeletal injuries in their workers' compensation system.

The medical literature and community considers that a treatment has become a standard of care when it has at least two to three Level I studies that can attest to the efficacy and safety of the procedure. Prolotherapy is very close to reaching this status. PRP, ASCI, and PSI still need to be researched and written about in the literature before they are viewed as standards of care.

How many procedures have you personally performed?

I have performed over 1,000 prolotherapy procedures a year since 2000.

I have performed more than 500 PSI procedures a year since 2006.

I have performed over 400 PRP procedures a year since 2007.

I performed fifty ASCI procedures in 2009. Each year this number rises. It was 120 in 2013.

GENERAL INFORMATION

What are the RIT procedures actually like?

They are similar to other orthopedic injection treatments in the following ways. The area of pathology is determined by physical examination and diagnostic testing. The area is marked and prepared with an approved preparation to sterilize the skin. Most doctors use an anesthetic superficially to reduce the discomfort of the procedure. The needle is placed in the pathologic location with or without guidance, and the treatment solution is injected. RIT can deliver injections to more locations and structures than typical orthopedic injections, which are limited to bursas, tendon sheaths, and joints. RIT procedures involve injecting liga-ment-stabilizing and joint capsule-stabilizing structures with proliferative (prolotherapy) or biologic (PRP and ASCI) solu-tions to increase the stability of the joint. Tendinopathic or torn tendons, as well as muscle tears, can be injected directly with a proliferative or biologic solution. Steroid injections delivered di-rectly into tendons and muscles can cause adverse effects, such as tendon ruptures and myonecrosis in muscles.

When using biologic treatments in RIT, most doctors guide their injections with ultrasound or x-ray guidance to make sure delivery of the cells is as accurate as possible to produce the de-sired healing effect. Most orthopedic injections are generally performed with "blind" technique.

What equipment do I need?

For all procedures, I highly recommend a hydraulic exam-ining table, both for your comfort and safety, as well as for the comfort of your patients. I strongly recommend investing in a good ultrasound machine, such as those manufactured by Gen-eral Electric, Sonosite, Terason, or Biosound. For PRP, you also need a proper centrifuge system. There are two different types of systems: one that separates out blood from the PRP prepara-tion, and one that doesn't. The "bloodless" centrifuge I now pre-fer is manufactured by EmCyte. "Blood-filled" PRP centrifuges are produced by companies including Harvest, Arteriocyte, An-gel, and Biomet. For ASCI, all of the aforementioned bedside centrifuge systems provide kits that can produce a concentrat-ed bone marrow stem cell preparation. How high-quality these systems are when it comes to actual cell counts doesn't come close to what we are getting with the Regenexx system. With the

Regenexx system, you additionally need a biologic safety closet or hood to prepare the cellular medicine samples for reinjection. For all of these procedures, you need the proper kits, solutions, syringes, and sterile equipment. You may also need proper state health agency certificates showing that you are in compliance with all state laws and regulations concerning the safe handling of human blood samples.

How do you introduce RIT treatments to patients?

First, I progress through all of the standard, conservative treatment options and the underused, but effective ancillary treatments I have already outlined in *Regenerative Healing*. If none of these have returned the patient to the level of functioning and pain management he desires, I explain the surgical options available to him. I also introduce the idea of regenerative injection treatments. I am careful to explain to patients that these treatments are not covered by insurance. I review with the patient my special consent forms for RIT treatments, which outline the possible benefits, risks, and complications. Depending on the severity of the disease and the patient's financial ability, I generally recommend prolotherapy first as the least expensive and most efficacious for mild disease. I recommend PRP, which is a moderately expensive treatment, for advancing stages of disease and stable cartilage injury. I recommend ASCI, which is the most costly, for severe disease. I tell patients there are informative video clips of these treatments, accompanied by brief explanations, on my website. I suggest that patients view these and then ask me any outstanding questions during their next appointment.

How would I answer a patient who wonders if RIT is painful or dangerous?

You can explain that the injections can cause some pain, but, properly done, this is minimal. Once the patient is numbed, most patients say that the treatment is mild to moderately painful to undergo. Patients tend to experience the procedure more as an obnoxious pressure than outright pain. However, some patients don't respond well to anesthetics and tend to feel pain more. There are some locations—like the inside of the knee, the outside of the hip, the palm side of the hand, or the bottom of the foot—that tend to be more sensitive to pain.

Check my website (www.drshiple.com) to see what a modern RIT treatment is actually like. Particularly note the excerpts from my PBS special about RIT. You can recommend these to your potential patients to give them a visual counterpoint to any negative material they may have seen on the Internet.

You can explain to patients that RIT procedures, according to Simon Dagenais, Ph.D., a researcher and chiropractor, are no more dangerous than any other in-office procedure performed in orthopedics.[13]

There are different ways to be trained in prolotherapy, and a doctor's training will impact the patient's perception of the procedure. I like to explain to patients that there is an "East Coast" and "West Coast" method of training. Practitioners of the West Coast method tend to use a more vigorous, blind injection technique requiring bigger needles. The physician has been trained to bang the tip of the needle on the bone to try to stimulate bleeding and, thus, healing. The early West Coast prolotherapists, such as Earl Gedney, D.O., Kent Pomeroy, M.D., and Milne Ongley, M.D., practiced and taught this way. This technique works well, but it can be more painful and may require a longer recovery time than the East Coast method. Ross Hauser, M.D., who was trained by Gus Hemwall, M.D., has videos online that show him performing prolotherapy with a rapid, jackhammer-like technique. Thomas Ravin, M.D., who was also trained by Dr. Hemwall, uses larger gauge needles and tends to perform his procedures this way. Don't get me wrong: Drs. Hauser and Ravin are excellent prolotherapists. They have successfully treated legions of patients. My point is simply that their technique differs from the East Coast one.

I and other practitioners of the East Coast method use a gentler technique to place the needle in the target area. Most use the smallest needle possible and mix some lidocaine with the dextrose. We generally use pre-treatment anesthesia with subcutaneous blebs of lidocaine over the needle entry point. Some practitioners of both methods use ultrasound guidance when necessary. Particularly in complex procedures, ultrasound can improve accuracy and minimize the amount of solution necessary. Less solution can mean less discomfort. I believe that the less pain a patient experiences and the shorter his recovery time, the more likely he will be to return for subsequent treatments and thus have a successful healing experience. Some doctors call the East Coast method the "Hackett-Hemwall" method.

Who is not a candidate for RIT?

Patients who have end-stage disease, such as the complete UCL tear of the elbow often seen in overhead-throwing athletes, are not good candidates. In this instance, the patient should undergo an MR arthrogram to document the extent to which the dye is leaking through the torn ligament. The UCL should be surgically repaired in such a case.

Patients who are on drugs that prevent their immune systems from reacting to RIT, such as etanercept (Enbrel), which is a biologic, rheumatoid medication, are also not good candidates. Nor are patients who are immune compromised due to disease or other reasons. Patients who cannot undergo mildly to moderately painful treatments, cannot take the time to heal, or cannot afford the out-of-pocket expense should also seek other treatments.

Does age affect RIT recovery results?

The very old and those with otherwise heavily diseased or degenerated tissue will have a harder time healing than those with otherwise healthy tissue. Although doctors are generally reluctant to treat the very young with any musculoskeletal injection therapy, when RIT is indicated, the young usually heal very well. I have treated RIT patients as young as nine years old with excellent results.

Can RIT help rheumatoid arthritis?

I have successfully treated some cases. However, if the patient is on a biologic medication that interferes with his immune system, prolotherapy will not work. PRP might. If a rheumatoid arthritis patient has one joint that is inflamed, but his disease is otherwise well-controlled by his medication regimen, using PRP can be a good strategy to try to help get the patient's symptoms under control. However, a trial of a small-dose corticosteroid injection may help his pain calm down as well.

Does RIT interfere with other medication, or vice-versa?

Other medications can interfere with RIT. NSAIDs and steroids are particularly harmful to the full healing potential of RIT.

With stem cell treatments, many medications can interfere with MSCs' ability to survive and grow. A current list of these medications is included in Chapter Thirteen.

HOW TO PROCEED WITH TRAINING
IF YOU ARE INTERESTED

Where can I train to do prolotherapy procedures?
There are a number of associations that offer training courses: the American Association of Orthopaedic Medicine (AAOM), the Hackett-Hemwall Foundation (HHF), the American Academy of Osteopathy (AAO), and the American Osteopathic Association of Prolotherapy Regenerative Medicine (AOAPRM). To be thoroughly trained, I recommend physicians attend an initial training course, at least one extended international training course, several weekend courses, and a yearly meeting with at least one of these organizations. The extended training courses are often international service trips, during which physicians serve poor and underserved patients outside of the United States while being proctored one on one with an expert teacher. Some physicians who practice RIT are also willing to mentor other physicians who are in training.

Where can I be trained to do perineural superficial injections (PSI)?
The American Association of Orthopaedic Medicine (AAOM) and John Lyftogt, M.D., both offer specific training in this technique.

Where can I be trained to do platelet-rich plasma (PRP) and adult autologous stem cell (ASCI) procedures?

There is one injection philosophy that contends that wherever a prolotherapy injection can be placed, so can a PRP injection. Consequently, the well-trained prolotherapist could conceivably perform PRP injections. However, since the volume of PRP obtained for a treatment is limited, it is advantageous for doctors performing this technique to also be trained in high-resolution ultrasound or C-arm fluoroscopic guidance. Additional training in PRP is available from the American Association of Orthopaedic Medicine (AAOM), the American Osteopathic Association of Prolotherapy Regenerative Medicine (AOAPRM), BlueTail Regenerative Therapeutics, and Steven Sampson, D.O., who is part of the Orthohealing Center. These organizations will train you in the actual PRP procedure, as well as various preparation techniques. Additional training in PRP preparation techniques is also available from the companies that make the centrifuges used in the procedure.

As with prolotherapy, I recommend physicians attend an initial training course, at least one other course each year on these techniques, and a yearly meeting with at least one of the training organizations. Since these techniques are complex and evolving, I also recommend that doctors practicing them visit other clinics, receive mentoring from other doctors, collaborate with colleagues, and keep up with journal articles.

See the Resources section at the back of the book for more information on the organizations above.

How long would the training take?

Depending on the amount of free or not-so-free time you have, anywhere from one to several years.

How would doing RIT affect my practice?

If your practice currently consists of evaluations, medication management, and referrals to specialists, learning interventional orthopedics and RIT would allow you to do in-office procedures in addition to your other work. It would also give you a variety of new ways in which you could help your patients heal or manage their orthopedic conditions. In terms of effects on business, it could substantially impact your reimbursements from insurance. Remember that many aspects of RIT are not covered by insurance. This means you will need to be comfortable explaining to patients that they will need to pay out of pocket.

At the time of writing, the average charge for a prolotherapy treatment in the U.S. ranges from $100–600 for a fifteen- to sixty-minute treatment. The range of charges for PRP is between $400 and $2,000. The range of cost of PSI is between $100 and $600. ASCI in the U.S. ranges from $1,000–$20,000, depending on the sophistication and extent of the treatment, and what is being treated.

More specifics about the business aspects of RIT and your practice will be covered in any training course you take.

How can I learn more about the new paradigm, prolotherapy, PSI, PRP, and ASCI?

For specific visual descriptions of each procedure, refer to the appropriate section of my website. To read more about any of these procedures, refer to the Recommended Reading section at the back of the book. Articles are listed both by procedure and specific problem areas.

POLITICS AND FINANCES

If you just work with prolotherapy, PRP, and PSI correctly and with sufficient training, you are working in as safe and legal a territory as in other cutting-edge fields of medicine. The RIT method that is mired in politics is ASCI.

What is the history of these politics?

The FDA gave itself regulatory power to make sure embryonic stem cells were being used safely, ethically, and to help treat certain conditions that had no cure. When scientists realized how many hurdles had to be overcome to work within the FDA's framework, combined with federal funding restrictions on this research, they started to explore autologous stem cells, which come from the patient's own tissue. Autologous stem cells are much safer because there is no chance of rejection by the body, and because there is no chance of transmitting a genetic disease or condition. They proved as efficacious as embryonic stem cells for most conditions, and are far cheaper to use for research and for clinical treatments. When the FDA realized scientists and physicians were using autologous stem cells in scientific studies and experimental treatments, they began to create a whole new set of rules that researchers now have to follow.

A concept that appears to guide their rules is that if a stem cell or any cell is "manipulated" more than a little bit, the cell is no longer considered a "native cell." It has now turned into something else, which they consider a drug. An example is that if fat has been extracted and separated from the blood that comes with it, it is minimally manipulated and therefore is permitted to be used in certain circumstances in stem cell work. Specifically, doctors can use raw fat as a graft to which stem cells can adhere while they are preparing to activate and help heal the surrounding tissue. However, if a physician uses the stromal vascular fraction (SVF) with a chemical to digest the raw fat and make the stem cells readily available to the target tissue, he has changed the fat tissue more than a minimal amount. Consequently, he has broken the minimal manipulation FDA rule.[17] He can be subject to fines, imprisonment, and losing his license to practice medicine. Many of my patients find it upsetting that a person's own tissue can be classified as a drug and regulated by the federal government.

The FDA also determined that the tissue a doctor extracts from a patient's body cannot be put in an area of the body where it would not naturally be found. This ruling is called the non-homologous use rule. So if a plastic surgeon takes abdominal fat and transfers it to the subcutaneous fat in the face, this is a homologous use of the transferred fat graft. However, if a physician were to transfer the fat to a tissue that does not normally have fat in it, then he would have broken this FDA rule, which is also a punishable offense.

In another ruling, the FDA made it illegal for a doctor to grow bone marrow stem cells or fat-derived stem cells in culture.[18] That means when a doctor in the United States harvests stem cells, he may get hundreds of thousands of usable mesenchymal stem cells from a patient's bone marrow sample. In countries where it is legal to grow stem cells in a lab, a culture can yield tens or hundreds of millions of MSCs per milliliter. This allows doctors in those countries to potentially treat more severe disease and/or larger areas more effectively with a single treatment.

While the FDA does have a duty to protect citizens from unsafe drugs and to make sure drugs are safely distributed across state lines, the physicians who practice cellular medicine in the U.S. question the aforementioned rulings. Should the FDA be involved in regulating a patient's tissue and how I decide to use it in the practice of medicine? Or is that between my patient and me? The FDA did not step in and regulate in-vitro fertilization. In this procedure, a doctor takes a woman's embryo and surgically transfers a man's sperm, then implants it into a uterus to create a human being. If this form of tissue transfer is legal, why does the FDA want to regulate the use of a person's bone marrow or fat?

Those of us who practice ASCI believe our treatments are rendered inviolable by the fact that the Food, Drug, Cosmetic Act and the courts have long protected the doctor–patient relationship from overreaching arms of our government. When I ask a patient to sign a consent form, I explain that these treatments are still experimental. I explain the current standard of care in our community, such as joint replacement or other surgery. I explain what we know and what we don't know. I explain the known risks and side effects of the treatments I am performing. It then becomes the patient's decision whether he wants me to use his cells, his own tissue to treat the orthopedic injury or disease in question. If the patient consents to have me perform the procedure to try to help them, according to the Food, Drug, Cosmetic Act, that is between my patient and me. Until the FDA became involved, the doctor-patient relationship was a sacred one with which no government agency could interfere.

If a doctor accidentally harmed a patient or an unforeseen

side effect occurred, the patient could report the doctor to the state board of medicine and could sue for damages he sustained. This is the safeguard in our medical system that ensures a doctor keeps within reasonable, responsible rules of medicine.

What is the financial reality of the stem cell debate?

Follow the money. This is where fortunes will be made that will make the Viagra pharmaceutical gold mine look like peanuts. Everyone wants to be the one to capture this pot of gold.

Big pharmaceutical companies stand to make billions in the untapped stem cell market if stem cells are classified as a drug. The pharmaceutical industry makes its money by taking a drug and mass-producing it, and then selling it across state lines. The reason big pharmaceutical companies cannot make a profit in the in-vitro fertilization (IVF) market is because IVF is a surgical procedure performed on one patient at a time. There is no part of the procedure that can be reproduced millions and millions of times and sold as a drug. The only money to be made with in-vitro fertilization goes to the hospitals and physicians who perform the procedure individually, one patient at a time.

In the stem cell market, the pharmaceutical companies own cell-line therapies, where an individual stem cell is reproduced millions and millions of times to create a cell culture that can be sold to doctors and hospitals to treat various medical and orthopedic conditions. This is where the pharmaceutical industry can realize a large return on its research investment if all stem cell therapies are sold this way. The beauty of autologous stem cell work is that each patient becomes the source for his own stem cells, making it far safer and less expensive because the pharmaceutical industry is taken out of the equation.

When a pharmaceutical company applies for a new drug license, its cost to bring a new drug to market can be as much as $800 million.[19] Because of the FDA's rulings considering each person's stem cells to be a drug, it could cost patients and physicians millions per patient to get a drug license through the FDA, that would make an individual's fat-derived or cultured stem cell treatment legal. Obviously, this makes these processes totally unfeasible. So unless a doctor is performing fat-derived stem cell experiments under an Investigational New Drug (IND) license with the FDA and has a research institutional review board registered with the FDA, these treatments are illegal in the United States. There are currently forty FDA-approved studies in the United States, a few of which deal with orthopedic disease.

Without a major policy shift, some very promising treatments for those suffering from arthritis and other degenerative diseases will remain unavailable to people in this country, while legitimate stem cell advances are progressing in other countries at breakneck speed, leaving the United States in the proverbial stem cell-market dust.

FREQUENTLY ASKED QUESTIONS

Following are some of the questions I am most frequently asked by my patients, and potential patients, along with the answers I give them. While some of these questions are about prolotherapy, PRP and PSI, most are about adult autologous stem cell injections (ASCI). These should prove helpful to you in talking with your patients. If a patient wants me to review his individual case, I prefer he make an appointment for a face-to-face consultation. If he lives far away from my office, I will set up a telephone case review, after he has submitted the proper paperwork and tests to me. Final treatment planning and further costs for treatment are discussed during these times.

1. **Can a stem cell injection grow your cartilage back in your bone-on-bone degenerative arthritic joint?** Probably not yet. We have a few cases with repeat MRI data that have shown regeneration of some surface cartilage. At least one patient who has had four stem cell treatments in the last three years has definitely shown significant regeneration of her surface cartilage on repeat MRI imaging. It may be that with repeated stem cell injections, we can expect to see more and more cartilage regeneration. This is a topic for future research we intend to undertake at Regenexx. For those of you with focal cartilage defects, read on.

2. **Why do patients report they are doing so well if they are not growing their cartilage back?** The answer is that we don't know exactly. We are probably changing the cellular and chemical composition of the joint for an extended time period. We know the arthritic joint is a hostile environment for the continued survival of already degenerating cartilage. We know that injecting good growth factors in an arthritic joint improves this chemical environment for a while. How long is a while? The Filardo PRP study showed clinical improvement in arthritis of the knee with a series of three PRP injections over nine months.[20] According to Regenexx data, with same-day stem cell procedure, patients average eighteen months of relief with one to two series of these treatments. For arthritis of the knee and hip, the range of relief goes from six months to five years for one to two series of stem cell injections.

3. **What are my chances of getting good pain relief if I have bone-on-bone arthritis of the knee or hip?** The answer is about 60 percent of patients with advanced arthritis get to the point where they experience at least 50 percent pain relief. This is the clinical criteria for a good outcome in most orthopedic surgery research. Anecdotally, the addition of a fat graft to the bone marrow treatment seems to increase the odds of getting good pain relief up to about 80 percent. To confirm this, we at Regenexx are planning on conducting a study to determine whether this observation is true or not.

4. **What if I have less severe arthritis? Are my chances to experience a good outcome with stem cell injections improved?** Yes, definitely. We see better results that last longer if we can intervene at an earlier stage in the degenerative process. The eight years of Regenexx data does seem to support this observation.

5. **How much better are the odds with less severe arthritis?** Eighty percent of patients are happy at the end of their treatment (without fat grafting) and report that they would undergo the treatment again and recommend it to friends and family.

6. **What if I have a torn labrum or torn meniscus or a chondral lesion in my joint?** The answer to this question is "it depends." If the lesion is very large and unstable, we probably cannot help you without surgical repair or removal. However, most of the time, the lesions are not that big. If the lesion is an unstable, herniated knee meniscus tear, for instance, we have a treatment protocol aimed at stabilizing the meniscus and healing the tear after the cells are inject-

ed on site. The joint is then braced for six to twelve weeks to help the meniscus heal in the right position. The most exciting results I have seen are on focal chondral lesions in younger adult and adolescent athletes. We are seeing excellent filling in of these smaller cartilage lesions and the avoidance of microfracture surgery. In my opinion, if faced with a decision to undergo stem cell injections or have surgery, surgery should only be a treatment of last resort.

7. **How many treatments are required to give me the best outcome attainable for my problem?** First of all, a stem cell treatment consists of three separate treatments:

A. Pre-treatment consists of a hypertonic dextrose solution or a platelet lysate injected in your joint to calm it down and prepare it for the stem cell injection the following week. It is much more advantageous for the stem cells to be injected into a joint that is not so inflamed. Any unstable ligaments are pre-treated as well to provide the joint with a more stable support system and to prepare the joint for the stem cell injections. This treatment, including the initial consultation, takes one to one-and-a-half hours to complete.

B. Stem Cell Day occurs one week after the pre-treatment. During this treatment, you return for the bone marrow aspiration. If needed, we will also perform a mini-liposuction to prepare a fat graft. In addition, your blood is drawn for a stem cell plasma preparation. Then, depending on your clinical problem, the cells are injected into the joint and cartilage lesions inside the joint, and also into the supporting ligaments and tendons if needed. This treatment takes two to two-and-a-half hours to complete.

C. Post-treatment injection is performed with a platelet-rich plasma treatment into the joint, or any place the stem cells were injected, to help them stay on site. This keeps them working a little longer before they are done. This treatment takes up to an hour to complete.

The more severe the orthopedic problem, the greater the chance of needing more than one treatment to attain the pain relief and healing we are hoping you will achieve. With that said, in the last year, I have only had to retreat three patients to help them reach their treatment goals. Only two patients have failed their treatment and been sent to orthopedic surgery. What constitutes a treatment failure? The patient exhibits no clinical improvement by the three-month mark after treatment.

8. **How many stem cell treatments and other cellular medicine treatments have you performed?** At the time of this writing in 2013, I perform approximately one to two stem cell cases a week and ten to twenty PRP cases a week. I also do ten to twenty prolotherapy cases a week. I perform approximately six to ten interventional spine cases a week. I've been performing stem cell treatments for more than four years, PRP for more than five years, spine injections for seven years, and prolotherapy for thirteen years. Almost all of my injections are either guided with C-arm fluoroscopy or with high-resolution ultrasound technology or both.

9. **Where can I find research on stem cell treatments?** You may find a list of articles under the ASCI section of the recommended reading list in this book. You can also consult my website, www.drshiple.com, or the Regenexx website, www.regenexx.com.

10. **What kind of problems can be treated?** Stem cell injections can treat degenerative arthritis of the shoulder, elbow, wrist and hands, as well as the hip, spine, knee, ankle and foot. They are also used for most types of ligament sprains, tendon tears without significant retraction, certain types of meniscal and labral tears, and certain size chondral lesions. They are also helpful to treat avascular necrosis of the end of the bones in joints, as well as certain bones in the foot and wrist. Stem cell injections are also used for certain types of non-union fractures.

11. **Can non-musculoskeletal medical conditions be treated with stem cells?** The Regenexx network does not offer stem cell treatments for medical conditions at this time. This includes spinal cord injury or disease.

12. **What are the risks, complications and side effects of a cellular medicine treatment?** Any time a needle is placed into the human body there is a chance of bleeding, bruising, pain, infection, and nerve injury.

    A. When performing the procedure with ultrasound or x-ray guidance the risk of hitting a large blood vessel that could cause excessive bruising or bleeding is much less than when the treatments are performed without guidance. With that said, we expect our patients to experience some bruising after a treatment. This usually clears up in a week or two even after liposuction and bone marrow aspirations, which use larger than normal needles.

    B. The pain involved is related to the needle procedure and then, after the procedure, by the initial inflammation produced in the injected tissue by the treatment.

The pain is minimized during the procedure when possible with superficial injections of lidocaine. Sometimes the anesthesia can be injected closer to the target tissue to minimize the effect of the procedure pain. We also employ regional anesthesia blocks to help the patient feel minimal pain when his joint is being treated. The pain following a procedure is treated with narcotic pain medication for a few days to a few weeks, depending on what area was treated and the patient's tolerance to pain.

C. Although I have not experienced an infection in my patients in close to twenty years of practice, the chance of suffering an infection from a needle-based procedure is 1 in 50,000 for a joint-based injection. We take meticulous care in our skin preparation and follow all injection guidelines, such as those produced by the ISIS organization.

D. Nerve injury is a rare occurrence in injection work, especially when performed with guidance. What patients need to understand is that it is not normal or expected to hit a nerve during regenerative injection work. If you ever feel an electric shock going down the limb or pins and needles during an injection, let your doctor know immediately so the needle can be redirected. The good thing is that even if the nerve is touched and injected with cells or dextrose, nerves usually recover very quickly and completely. The risk of permanent injury to nerves when inadvertently injected by anesthesiologists performing regional anesthesia in the operating room setting is 1 in 90,000.

13. **Does the bone marrow draw hurt?** Despite common belief, it is actually much less painful than most people think. Eighty-three percent of Regenexx patients reported in a survey that the bone marrow draw was much less painful than they anticipated, and they would return for a repeat treatment without hesitation.

14. **What about the risk of stem cells causing tumors to form at the injection site?** This is an excellent question, and one based on fact. However, there is no report of a tumor growing in an orthopedically treated area where the patient's own cells were injected. Tumor growth is a real possibility in two circumstances:

    A. In embryonic stem cell work, where the genetic makeup of another human being is injected into your body. The genetic influence and triggers that may cause the stem cells to mutate or form a tumor in the future is a real risk one assumes when receiving embryonic or any autogenic stem cells from another human being.

    B. In culture-expanded stem cells, which carry the risk of being grown too long or of being put through too many passages in culture. The risk here is the more passages a stem cell is passed through, the more chances the stem cell can mutate into a tumor cell that could go unrecognized and be implanted into the host patient, thus putting him at risk of developing a tumor. At the time of this writing in 2013, it is illegal to culture expand stem cells in the United States, so this should never happen if the stem cells are being handled and procedures performed according to FDA rules. With that said, Regenexx has the ability to culture expand a patient's stem cells in the Cayman Island Regenexx Clinic. In that lab, they never run a patient's stem cells through more than five stem cell passages (which is the maximum amount allowed by protocol before the risk of mutations start to be seen). Before they are injected into the patient, the patient's grown stem cells are sent back to the lab in the United States to make sure there is no sign or evidence of tumor cells.

15. **Have you ever made someone worse with your cellular medicine treatment?** No, I have not. However, there were two patients who at the time I worried I may have made worse with their extensive stem cell treatments. Both had extensive instability along with terrible cartilage lesions and/or severe arthritis. After they completed their stem cell treatments, they both had dramatic increases in their stability. In both cases, a nearby unstable joint that was not treated suddenly became painful. Upon follow up and recognition of the problem, the unstable joint was treated twice and each patients' newfound pain issue cleared up.

16. **Are the treatments covered by insurance, Medicare, worker's compensation, auto accident insurance?**

    A. No, not at this time. Stem cell use is still very experimental, and third party payers have very well-defined non-coverage policies on their web sites. It is usually called autologous blood-based therapies, which covers PRP and stem cell injections. They also have a section on prolotherapy not being covered. They all cite the reason as there not being enough research evidence to show that these treatments work in large populations.

    B. We do not and will not provide any codes for a patient

to try to submit the CPT codes to their insurance company for reimbursement for the following two reasons.

- The government has not developed any CPT codes for stem cell treatments.
- If a practice gives the codes out that are available (for instance, the temporary code for PRP), and you successfully can get your plan to reimburse you, in doing so you just caused your physician to commit insurance fraud. He signed a contract with your insurance company stating he agreed not to charge your payer for non-covered services. This can result in the physician losing his contract with the insurance company, paying back all money received from patients who were charged out-of-pocket for previous procedures, and also being heavily fined. There is no fighting this at the time of writing. It has happened to me and to others.

17. **How does each type of regenerative injection treatment compare to the others?** I like my patients to think of these treatment options on a continuum of care spectrum, starting with the mildest, easiest, cheapest at the low end and moving to the most expensive, sophisticated, strongest on the high end of the spectrum.

A. Prolotherapy is the safest, cheapest, and most effective place to start for milder disease. The younger the patient, the better it works. With that said, it still can help in more advanced disease and in patients of advanced age, but the chance of significant improvement falls with severity and age. It can take three to six prolotherapy treatments to heal or manage most orthopedic conditions, with a range of one to ten.

B. PRP is probably equal to two to three prolotherapy treatments, but it can cost two to three times more than a prolotherapy treatment. I generally prefer to use it for more unstable ligament tears, larger tendon tears, more advanced cartilage lesions and more advanced arthritis. It can take two to three treatments, with a range of one to five to heal or manage most orthopedic conditions that I treat.

C. Stem cells are reserved for the worst tendon disease, ligament tears, cartilage lesions, and even more advanced arthritis. It also can attain in one treatment in a milder case what two to three PRP treatments can achieve. It may be more cost-effective to go right to a stem cell treatment plan for someone with a limit to the amount of time he can commit to his healing schedule. This is especially true for someone traveling a great distance to come in for treatment. The other advantage is that the length of symptom relief a patient usually experiences from a stem cell treatment may be two to three times that of a series of PRP treatments.

18. **What are the out-of-pocket costs at the time of writing for the various treatment options I offer my patients?**

A. Prolotherapy costs a minimum of $150 for one ultrasound-guided injection in my clinic. The more sites injected, the more time and materials it takes to complete the treatment. Therefore, the more expensive it is. Costs range from $150–$600 to treat any given area or region. This includes ultrasound guidance in most scenarios. Actual costs will be determined after a full evaluation of a patient's problem with a history, physical examination, diagnostic ultrasound evaluation and review of any pertinent diagnostic films and other test results.

B. PRP treatments range from $750 for a small joint to $1,100 for a large region, like a sports hernia. This includes ultrasound examination each time a treatment is performed, ultrasound guidance, a PRP kit, preparation of the PRP, a platelet count in our automatic platelet counter, and injection of the PRP to all necessary sites to complete the treatment plan.

C. Fat grafting is an additional $1,000–$2,000 to perform the mini-liposuction, spin the fat sample to separate the fat from the blood and oil and prepare the fat for implantation, as well as to perform the injection with ultrasound guidance.

D. A Regenexx stem cell injection at this time costs $4,275 for a single joint or region. This includes performing the bone marrow aspiration and preparing the bone marrow concentrate and injecting the cells back into the joint or tendon as part of the plan of care. This includes counting cells on an automatic stem cell counter as well as a research fee, as all of my patients are required to enroll in our Regenexx patient registry so researchers back at the home office can follow outcomes, including any complications or side effects that may occur. This data will also serve as a rich database to conduct clinical research on the outcomes patients experience. Our research is self-funded. There are no pharmaceutical companies or organizations from other industries that are going to help us with the cost to fund the research that is desperately needed to prove whether stem cells are any better than surgery or a steroid shot. The cost for the registry is $150 dollars per patient. It is factored into the cost of the stem cell treatment. This cost helps cover the salaries of the researchers at the home office. The research fee is paid one time for each joint during the first treatment, and covers that joint until your treatment is finished. If another joint at another time is treated the research fee will be charged again.

19. **Do you offer a payment plan for the treatments above?** No, we do not. Payment is expected at the time of treatment by credit card, check, or cash.

20. **How far out are you scheduling stem cell procedures?** In early 2013, it takes about two to three months to get on the schedule. This also gives patients adequate time to prepare for their treatment.

21. **Why not just get surgery to fix my problem?** Surgery is always an option patients are faced with when they suffer from severe arthritis, a cartilage tear, a severe ligament tear or a tendon tear. Surgery is the treatment of choice in my community for badly torn cartilage and bone-on-bone arthritis. However, we all know friends and loved ones who didn't have the outcome they were hoping for after their surgery. Stem cell injections help many of my patients avoid surgery, but not all of them. Some are simply too far-gone, and I tell them so when we discuss their case. Joint replacement surgery is 90 percent successful, but only 70 percent of patients are satisfied with their outcomes. I see a lot of these 30 percent dissatisfied patients in my practice. They wonder what went wrong, and how I can help them now after their surgery. They warn their loved ones

to do anything they can to avoid their fate. That's why I began to offer these experimental procedures to my patients. The bottom line is, the risk of putting your cells into your orthopedic problem area is very low. The upside, which is significant in most of my patients' cases, is the potential to avoid the surgery they would otherwise face. If you can afford the treatment, you understand your chances, and you are willing to accept the risks, complications and benefits, then consider getting a stem cell treatment. I would especially warn patients who are facing a joint replacement who are younger than sixty, or those who have a torn meniscus in their knee and also have arthritis, that the risk of having complications resulting in further surgery and chronic pain are significantly high.

22. **What about stem cells for a spine condition?** Stem cells and PRP are being used in spine conditions with questionable results. Regenexx tried using the same-day stem cell procedure into degenerated, painful discs, and it was somewhat successful. However, they have been able to get better pain relief and regeneration of the disc with cultured stem cell treatments at the Cayman Islands Stem Cell Center. We have nothing to offer our end-stage spinal stenosis patients other than standard interventional spine treatments. We do have some options for patients with arthritis in a facet joint and nerves that are irritated by a herniated disc. Traditionally, pain doctors inject high-dose steroids around the nerve or into the joints. These only have a temporary effect. Putting PRP into the arthritic joints with C-arm fluoroscopic guidance is helping many of my patients avoid the radio frequency ablation where

the nerves to the painful facet joint have to be burned with radiofrequency heat energy every year or so to help them attain pain relief. We can also inject a patient's lysate with an ultra low dose of steroid to help calm the inflamed nerve near a damaged disc with as much pain relief as a regular steroid shot. This minimizes the risk of the patient getting too much steroids in a year. I have been invited to be part of a new spinal disc restoration study in 2013. An experimental drug cocktail, under research for the last ten years, will be injected into degenerated, painful discs after first performing a discogram procedure to confirm whether the disc in question is causing the patient's pain. This is an exciting new frontier in interventional spine medicine that might make spinal fusion surgery a rare event in medicine.

23. **What about stem cells for bone fractures?** Stem cells in bone fractures already have an important role in orthopedics. Non-unions can finally heal if concentrated bone marrow stem cells are injected directly into the fracture site and stabilized with another period of immobilization. Also well established is the role of concentrated bone marrow injections into bones that have suffered avascular necrosis or osteonecrosis, otherwise known as death of the bone. AVN of the hip, knee and ankle are areas where we are seeing a successful alternative to surgical drilling to try to re-establish blood flow and healing in the dying bone. The process involves drilling a hole into the bone with AVN using C-arm fluoroscopic guidance and a sterile surgical drill bit and cannula. Then some radiopaque dye is injected into the diseased bone to confirm the needle is in the right spot. Once confirmation of the dye being

in the right area is seen, a mixture of concentrated bone marrow and some platelets are injected into the damaged area. The results are better than the classic surgical procedure of core decompression. A French orthopedic surgeon, Philippe Hernigou, M.D., has pioneered this work since the 1990s and has shown significant improvement over surgery. Patients with stage 1 and 2 AVN in the hip can expect about a 90 percent success rate with this stem cell procedure, and patients with stage 3 AVN of the hip, can expect 70–80 percent success, while those with stage 4 AVN can expect only 60-plus percent success.

24. **What can a patient do to help prepare for a stem cell treatment?** In Chapter Thirteen I recommend dietary changes that may help increase stem cell counts. There are supplements I recommend that may help prepare stem cells for the treatment. If you talk to a dozen doctors who perform stem cell treatments, you will get a dozen different answers on what you can and should be doing to prepare for a stem cell treatment. There really is only scant data on what if anything we can do to most effectively help prepare for a stem cell treatment. Most of this is theory at this point, or data that has been collected from university animal studies and extrapolated to humans. At Regenexx they are starting to study which supplements help or hurt stem cells grow in culture. For instance, vitamin D3 helps stem cells grow, much like adding Miracle Grow to tomato plants. Much more on this will be forthcoming in the future. Regenexx has also figured out a list of medicines that prevent stem cells from expanding in culture. This list seems to keep growing. It is also included in Chapter

Thirteen. In addition, it turns out that strength training can also help our stem cell numbers. For example, exercising in the pool to try to get some muscular development helps our stem cell numbers increase. This may be impossible for some patients, but any increase in strength can only help you prepare for your treatment.

25. **Can I talk to someone who has undergone a stem cell treatment?** Please check this book, my website (www.drshiple.com) or the Regenexx website for a list of patient testimonials regarding your area of concern.

26. **What if the patient doesn't have a recent MRI?** If an MRI is more than one year old or if the patient's condition has changed for the worse, we suggest you ask his treating physician or primary care physician for an updated MRI order, including a precertification, if required by his insurance plan. If I order the MRI, there is a high probability that it will not be covered by the patient's insurance, and he will be responsible for the MRI bill.

27. **What's the future for stem cell treatments in orthopedics?** Regenexx has a team of bioengineers and doctors that have new ideas they are bringing to the research department on a weekly basis. We are starting to figure out more sophisticated ways to deal with our patients' orthopedic problems that will change the specialty of orthopedics. Interventional cardiology was developed after cardiothoracic surgery to create minimally invasive catheter procedures to avoid open-heart surgery. We are developing interventional orthopedics, which are now office-based minimally invasive needle procedures to replace some orthopedic surgery procedures commonly done in the hospital.

28. **Are stem cell injections legal?** Yes. The use of your own tissue to treat a medical problem in your body is legal if doctors follow certain rules and regulations developed by the FDA. With that said, culture-expanding stem cells and creating a stromal vascular fraction stem cell solution from raw fat has been outlawed by the FDA as early as December of 2011. As long as the procedure is performed on the same day in the same clinic where the cells were harvested, we are operating within the guidelines and rules laid out by the FDA.

29. **Are stem cell injections approved by the FDA to treat orthopedic conditions we routinely treat?** The answer is no, they are not. The FDA does not approve treatments of disease. They approve medicines and devices used to treat patients. They are charged to protect the public from the harmful use of devices—such as surgical instruments or centrifuges that spin your cells—from ever reaching the doctor's office or hospital where patients are treated. They are also charged to make sure the medicine supply a doctor uses to treat his patients is safe and is transported safely across state lines.

30. **Why does the FDA have legal jurisdiction over cells?** That is a great question. The FDA was given regulatory power over tissues when it determined if a stem cell, or any tissue for that matter, was altered enough in preparation to treat a human being's disease or injury, it was no longer that person's cell. It had turned into a drug that the FDA has control over to make sure no harm can occur to the patient being treated by his own tissue, or drug, depending on your view point.

CONCLUSION

I hope that fifty years from now people will look back at the current model of medical care of injuries and degenerative diseases and wonder why we continued to use it when a new and more effective paradigm for helping patients had already been developed. If that scenario seems unlikely, remember that, until fifty years ago, people with arthritis or other disabling diseases had no viable alternatives to painkillers, canes, crutches, walking sticks, and wheelchairs. Medical science has made some enormous progress in the last five decades, and I believe we are now at a point where we can make even greater progress in the decades to come. The tools exist today to cure many "incurable" injuries and diseases. We simply need to introduce them to more patients and to get more physicians comfortable using them.

In the preceding pages, I have taken you with me on the incredible journey I began when I set out to find a treatment to help my own injuries, and those of the patients I cared for who seemed to be out of all options. Prior to RIT treatment, although they had followed the orders I or other specialists gave them, they were still unable to achieve the pain relief, function, and mobility they had enjoyed before they sustained injuries or musculoskeletal diseases. I have shared with you some amazing stories about people who wouldn't give up hope. Many of them found the help they were seeking through the new healing paradigm.

I have explained how people are injured, what happens physically at different stages of injury, and how the timing and type of medical care dispensed critically affects the outcome of an injury. You have learned that our musculoskeletal system is similar to an Erector Set. A loose fitting in one place affects the entire structure. Healing requires looking at the whole body and the whole person.

We have explored how an acute injury can become chronic,

The new fields of integrative and interventional orthopedic medicine brings together the fields of sports medicine and orthopedics in a new and positive way.

---

and what you must do to stop this process. I have given you a step-by-step guide for treating injuries well, so you or your loved ones won't join the ranks of people with chronic injuries and pain.

I have thoroughly explored the old-paradigm treatments most often used at this time, both their wonders and shortcomings. I have told you about underused methods that will help substantially in managing and healing injuries. Some of these are simple, "old time" remedies that have been lost in our societal rush to find the quickest fix. I have introduced you to the new fields of integrative and interventional orthopedic medicine, which bring together the fields of sports medicine and orthopedics in a new and positive way, creating many more alternatives to bridge the gap between conservative treatments and the necessity for surgery. I have told you how to find the best physicians, therapists, and practitioners of ancillary therapies.

We have looked at the innovative and amazing regenerative injection treatments that have brought relief to millions of patients. They include the sixty-year-old, "new" method of prolotherapy; the forty-year-old treatment of platelet-rich plasma; the newer and exciting treatments with autologous adult stem cell injections; and the promising, emerging field of perineural superficial injection treatment.

Through the willingness of some of my patients to share their experiences, I have given you numerous examples of how these treatments have helped to heal people with injuries of all kinds. I have also told you about patients with degenerative diseases who have halted or reversed the process of deterioration.

I have outlined the ground rules to optimize any RIT treatments, both in terms of things that will help and things to avoid. We have looked at medications which can hamper healing, and ones that can help. We have touched upon the importance of nutrition and the field of bioidentical hormone replacement. I have explained how to make the post-injection healing stages as comfortable and beneficial as possible.

We have looked together at some disturbing trends that could contribute to the out-of-control increase in the incidence of arthritis in the years to come. I have placed particular emphasis on physical overuse and overstress in the baby boomer population, as well as early specialization in sports among today's young people. I have discussed the fact that what you do to your body today can definitely affect how it functions in the years to come.

We have examined why people have to pay out of pocket for many of these new treatments, particularly regenerative injections. I have told you what steps are being taken to make these methods part of the accepted standard of care, and what you can do to help. I have answered the most frequently asked questions of physicians who are interested in providing these treatments for their patients.

Now it is your turn—whether you are a physician or patient—to take the knowledge you have gained and share it with others. Throughout the book, I have urged patients to become medically responsible individuals. This means they will be careful in selecting the physicians who treat them. They won't be reticent about telling their doctor their injury story or asking relevant questions

---

Now it is your turn—whether you are a physician or patient—to take the knowledge you have gained and share it with others.

---

about their care.

One of the questions they should ask their doctors is, "Why don't you offer me the new-paradigm treatments?" Another is, "Can you examine me with ultrasound and offer me regenerative injection techniques?" If the answer is negative, they might question the philosophy and practices of the doctor who isn't willing to treat patients with every reasonable treatment available.

I hope that many of the doctors reading this book will learn about these new techniques and get the training to do them well and offer them to their patients. I know that doing so has made me a much more competent physician, and one who knows I can offer my patients all reasonable, safe methods available to relieve them of their pain and suffering.

Patients, I hope never to hear of anyone who has read this book wearing his or her orthotics upside down, or having surgery before it is necessary to do so. Be choosey in selecting practitioners. Continue to educate yourself to be your own, your children's, your friend's medical advocate. In the current medical climate, everyone needs someone to help him or her hear clearly and understand fully, particularly when he or she is ill or injured.

I urge you all to remain aware of the political scene surrounding these methods of treatment, and to let your opinions be heard. Tell your doctors and your representatives that you want these treatments to be available and reimbursable.

We stand at the dawn of a new day in the treatment of musculoskeletal injuries and illnesses. You, the interested, medically responsible patient and physician, will help to determine whether we reach the full potential regenerative healing offers for life.

RESOURCES

Brian J. Shiple, D.O.
The Center for Sports Medicine
905 West Sproul Road, Suite 106
Springfield, Pennsylvania
(484) 472-8812
www.drshiple.com

In his practice in Springfield, Pennsylvania, Dr. Shiple treats the broad spectrum of sports medicine injuries, from the acute to chronic injury stage. This includes sprains or tears of ligaments, tendons, and muscles. He treats some forms of acute and chronic cartilage injuries, including those to the hyaline (surface), the meniscal and/or labral cartilage of the knee, and the cartilage of the shoulder and hip. In addition, Dr. Shiple treats tendinopathy (chronically diseased tendons), acute stable bone fractures, and some chronic fractures (stress fractures or non-union fractures).

Dr. Shiple treats avascular necrosis or osteonecrosis (or death of the bone) of certain bones, such as the hip, knee, ankle, tarsal navicular, if he sees the patient before the bone collapses. He treats some form of nerve entrapment, including carpal tunnel syndrome and tarsal tunnel syndrome. He performs interventional spine procedures using C-arm fluoroscopic guidance. Included in these are epidurals, facet joint injections, sacroiliac joint injections, and certain ganglion blocks, which help treat and manage spinal injuries and pain.

Dr. Shiple uses diagnostic ultrasound, along with standard x-ray and MRI evaluations, to help diagnose his patients' injuries or diseases. He uses anesthetic blocks to help diagnose and treat some conditions, and corticosteroid injections cautiously and sparingly, where indicated. He is expert in the use of hypertonic dextrose prolotherapy, platelet-rich plasma, autologous fat grafting, and concentrated bone marrow. These help treat a broad range of mild to severe orthopedic injuries and diseases, allowing his patients to heal their condition, if possible, or better manage their disease if a total cure is not possible.

To contact Dr. Shiple's office for an appointment, phone the number above. To locate a physician who performs some of the new-paradigm treatments in your area, contact the websites of the organizations mentioned below.

To invite Dr. Shiple to give a keynote address, lecture, or workshop for your upcoming event, please contact his business manager, Eileen, at the number above.

ASSOCIATIONS

To locate a new-paradigm physician near you, contact the associations below. Each will have a list of doctors in your area who practice these forms of medicine.

American Academy of Osteopathy (AAO)
3500 DePauw Boulevard, Suite 1080
Indianapolis, IN. 46268
(317) 879-1881
www.academyofosteopathy.org

American Association for Orthopaedic Medicine (AAOM)
555 Waterview Lane
Ridgeway, CO. 81432
Physicians only may phone: (888) 687-1920
www.aaomed.org

American Osteopathic Association of Prolotherapy Regenerative Medicine (AOAPRM)
303 South Ingram Court
Middletown, DE. 19709
(302) 530-2489
www.acopms.com

BlueTail Regenerative Therapeutics
Locations in Missouri, Ohio, and Utah
www.bluetail.org

Hackett-Hemwall Foundation (HHF)
2532 Balden Street
Madison, WI. 53713
www.hacketthemwall.org

Regenexx
Toll-free in the United States: (888) 525-3005
www.regenexx.com

PHYSICIANS

The following is an alphabetical list of new-paradigm physicians who are mentioned in the book and/or with whom Dr. Shiple has worked.

UNITED STATES

Arthur Bartolozzi, M.D.
(888) ORTHO3B
www.aria3bortho.org

Tommy Bond, M.D., M.S.
TotalCare
1101 South College Road, Suite 201
Lafayette, LA. 70503
(337) 264-7209
www.totalcare-la.com

Mark S. Cantieri, D.O., FAAO
Corrective Care
3555 Park Place West, Suite 200
Mishawaka, IN. 46545
(574) 498-0944
www.correctivecare.com

Christopher J. Centeno, M.D.
Regenexx Centeno-Schultz Clinic
403 Summit Boulevard, Suite 201
Broomfield, CO. 80021
(303) 429-6448
www.centenoschultz.com

Thomas Clark, D.C.
MSKUS
1035 E. Vista Way, Suite 128
Vista, CA. 92084
(760) 940-8900
www.mskus.com

David Crane, M.D.
Crane Clinic Sports Medicine
12855 North Forty Drive
Walker Medical Building
Suite 380, North Tower
St. Louis, MO. 63141
(314) 434-7784
www.craneclinic.com

Bjorn C. J. Eek, M.D.
901 Campus Drive, Suite 310
Daly City, CA. 94015
(650) 755-0733
Or: 27 Peters Canyon Road
Irvine, CA. 92606
(949) 261-8975
www.spinaldiagnostics.com

Dr. Mayo Friedles, M.D.
3031 Javier Road, Suite 100
Fairfax, VA. 22031
(703) 560-8280
www.treatingpain.com

Brian C. Halpern, M.D.
Hospital for Special Surgery
535 East 70th Street
New York, N.Y. 10021
(212) 606-1329
www.hss.edu

Ronald W. Hanson, Jr., M.D.
Centeno-Schultz Clinic
403 Summit Blvd, Suite 201
Broomfield, CO. 80021
(303) 429-6448
info@centenoschultz.com
www.centenoschultz.com

Shawn Kerger, D.O.
Doctors' Hospital Family Practice
  Center
2030 Stringtown Road, Suite 300
Grove City, OH. 43123
(614) 544-0101
www.doctorsfp.com
www.ohiohealth.com

W. Ben Kibler, M.D., FACSM
Lexington Clinic Orthopedics-
  Sports Medicine Center
700 Bob-O-Link Drive
Lexington, KY. 40504
(859) 258-8575
www.lexingtonclinic.com

Andrew Kochan, M.D.
Kochan Institute for Healing Arts
  Research
4835 Van Nuys Boulevard,
  Suite 100
Sherman Oaks, CA. 91403
(818) 995-9331
www.healingartsresearch.org

Albert J. Kozar, D.O., FAOASM
Valley Sports Medicine and
Orthopedic Medicine
54 West Avon Road, Suite 202
Avon, CT. 06001
(860) 675-0357
www.jockdoctors.com

Allan Mishra, M.D.
Menlo Medical Clinic
1300 Crane Street
Menlo Park, CA. 94025
(650) 498-7949
www.allanmishra.com

Robert Monaco, M.D.
Rutgers University/Hale Center
1 Scarlet Knight Way
Piscataway, N.J. 08854
(732) 445-2091
www.rwjuh.edu

Larry Nassar, D.O.
MSU Sports Medicine
4660 South Hagadorn Road,
   Suite 420
East Lansing, MI. 48823
(517) 884-6100
www.sportsmed.msu.edu/pages/
   nassar

Carl Osborn, D.O.
3156 State Street
Medford, OR. 97504
(541) 773-9772
www.ventanawellness.com

George J. Pasquarello, D.O., FAAO
East Greenwich Spine and Sport
1351 South County Trail, Suite 100
East Greenwich, R.I. 02818
(401) 886-5907
www.egss.us

**Jeffrey Patterson, D.O., professor
of family medicine, University of
Wisconsin School of Medicine,
and President, Hackett-Hemwall
Foundation**
Northeast Family Medical Center
   of the University of Wisconsin
3209 Dryden Drive
Madison, WI. 53704
(608) 241-9020
www.fammed.wisc.edu/directory/
   74

David P. Rabago, M.D.
Northeast Family Medical Center
   of the University of Wisconsin
3209 Dryden Drive
Madison, WI. 53704
(608) 241-9020
www.fammed.wisc.edu/directory/
   3968

Thomas H. Ravin, M.D.
Val d'Isere Health Clinic
45 South Dahlia Street
Denver, CO. 80246
(303) 331-9339
www.tomravinmd.com

K. Dean Reeves, M.D.
4740 El Monte Street
Roeland Park, KS. 66205
(913) 362-1600
www.drreeves.com

Steven Sampson, D.O.
10780 Santa Monica Blvd, Suite 210
Los Angeles, CA. 90025
(310) 453-5404
www.orthohealing.com

Michael A. Scarpone, D.O.
4100 Johnson Road, Suite 208
Steubenville, OH. 43952
(740) 266-3866
www.trinityhealth.com

John R. Schultz, M.D.
Centeno-Schultz Clinic
403 Summit Boulevard, Suite 201
Broomfield, CO. 80021
(303) 429-6448
www.centenoschultz.com

Jay P. Shah, M.D.
Rehabilitation Medicine
  Department
National Institutes of Health
  Clinical Center
www.cc.nih.gov
Research only

Paul Tortland, D.O., FAOASM
Valley Sports Physicians &
  Orthopedic Medicine
54 West Avon Road, Suite 202
Avon, CT. 06001
(860) 675-0357
www.jockdoctors.com

George Yu, M.D.
Aegis Medical Associates
116 Defense Highway, Suite 200
Annapolis, MD. 21401
(410) 897-0540
www.totallyyu.com

INTERNATIONAL

Philippe Hernigou, M.D.
http://chu-mondor.aphp.fr

Jan Kersschot, M.D.
www.kersschot.com

Young Uck Kim, M.D., Ph.D.
www.shortdigit.com/intro/doctor.
  jsp

John Lyftogt, M.D.
j_lyftogt@extra.co.nz

Jean Paul Ouellette, M.D.
Orthopaedic Medicine Clinic
2555 St. Joseph Boulevard,
  Suite 206
Ottawa, Ontario K1C 1S6
Canada
(613) 824-4223
www.cproloc.ca

David C. Reid, M.D.
Glen Sather University of Alberta
  Sports Medicine Clinic
Level 2 Edmonton Clinic
11400 University Avenue
Edmonton, Alberta T6G 1Z1
Canada
(780) 492-4752
www.glensatherclinic.ualberta.ca

Gaston Andres Topol, M.D.
www.proloterapia.com.ar

Gerjo van Osch, Ph.D.
www.erasmusmc.nl

RECOMMENDED READING

The following articles and books have been of great value and inspiration to me in writing *Regenerative Healing for Life*.

GENERAL INFORMATION ON OLD- AND NEW-PARADIGM TREATMENTS

R. Bellamy. "Compensation Neurosis: Financial Reward for Illness as Nocebo." *Clinical Orthopaedics and Related Research*, 1997.

Mark Frankle and Joseph Borrelli. "The Effects of Testosterone Propionate and Methenolone Enanthate on the Healing of Humeral Osteotomies in the Wistar Rat." *Journal of Investigative Surgery*, 1990.

Matthew Herper. "The Truly Staggering Cost of Inventing New Drugs." *Forbes.com*, February 2, 2012. http://www.forbes.com/sites/matthewherper/2012/02/22/the-truly-staggering-cost-of-inventing-new-drugs-the-print-version.

Christopher McDougall. *Born to Run*. Alfred A. Knopf, 2009.

Robert Maigne, M.D. *Diagnosis and Treatment of Pain of Vertebral Origin, second edition*. CRC Press, 2005.

Daniel David Palmer. *The Chiropractor's Adjuster*. Portland Printing House, 1910.

James A. Porterfield, "Dynamic Stabilization of the Trunk." *Journal of Orthopedic and Sports Physical Therapy*, 1985.

David C. Reid. *Sports Injury Assessment and Rehabilitation.* Churchill Living-stone, 1991. (Not currently in print, but available used.)

Jay P. Shah and Elizabeth A. Gilliams. "Uncovering the Biochemical Milieu of Myofascial Trigger Points Using in Vivo Microdialysis: An Application of Mus-cle Pain Concepts to Myofascial Pain Syndrome," *Journal of Bodywork and Movement Therapies,* 2008.

M.A. Slatyer, et al. "A Randomized Controlled Trial of Piroxicam in the Man-agement of Acute Ankle Sprain in Australian Regular Army Recruits. The Ka-pooka Ankle Sprain Study." *American Journal of Sports Medicine,* 1997.

Andrew Taylor Still. *The Philosophy and Mechanical Principles of Osteopathy.* Hudson-Kimberly Publishing Company, 1902.

Janet G. Travell and David G. Simons. *Myofascial Pain and Dysfunction: The Trigger Point Manual, volumes 1 and 2, second edition.* Lippincott Williams & Wilkins, 1998.

S. Williams, et al. "Kinesio Taping in Treatment and Prevention of Sports Inju-ries: A Meta-analysis of the Evidence for Its Effectiveness." *Journal of Orthope-dic and Sports Physical Therapy,* 2012.

RISKS AND COMPLICATIONS ASSOCIATED WITH THE OLD PARADIGM

M.R. Carmont, et al. "Simultaneous Bilateral Achilles Tendon Ruptures Asso-ciated with Statin Medication Despite Regular Rock Climbing Exercise." *Phys-ical Therapy in Sport,* 2009.

Emil Loldrup Fosbøl, et al. "Cause-specific Cardiovascular Risk Associated with Nonsteroidal Anti-inflammatory Drugs among Healthy Individuals." *Cir-culation: Cardiovascular Quality and Outcomes,* 2010.

Mark M. Mikhael, et al. "Failure of Metal-on-metal Total Hip Arthroplasty Mimicking Hip Infection: A Report of Two Cases." *American Journal of Bone and Joint Surgery,* 2009.

P. Otruba, et al. "Treatment with Statins and Peripheral Neuropathy: Results of 36-Months a Prospective Clinical and Neurophysiological Follow-up." *Neuro Endocrinology Letters*, 2011.

J. F. Reynolds, et al. "Non-steroidal Anti-inflammatory Drugs Fail to Enhance Healing of Acute Hamstring Injuries Treated with Physiotherapy." *South African Medical Journal*, 1995.

ON PROLOTHERAPY

OVERVIEW

Donna Alderman. "Prolotherapy for Musculoskeletal Pain." *Practical Pain Management*, 2007.

Simon Dagenais, et al. "Intraligamentous Injection of Sclerosing Solutions (Prolotherapy) for Spinal Pain: A Critical Review of the Literature." *Spine Journal*, 2005.

Simon Dagenais, et al. "Side Effects and Adverse Events Related to Intraligamentous Injection of Sclerosing Solutions (Prolotherapy) for Back and Neck Pain: A Survey of Practitioners." *Archives of Physical Medicine and Rehabilitation*, 2006.

Gerald R. Harris. "Neural Therapy and Its Role in the Effective Treatment of Chronic Pain." *Practical Pain Management*, 2009.

Young Uck Kim. "Case Reports and Cost Analysis." A paper presented to the Anatomy, Diagnosis, and Treatment of Chronic Myofascial Pain with Prolotherapy Research symposium at the University of Wisconsin School of Medicine and Public Health, October 21–23, 2012.

David Rabago, et al. "A Systematic Review of Prolotherapy for Chronic Musculoskeletal Pain." *Clinical Journal of Sports Medicine*, 2005.

Thomas H. Ravin, Mark S. Cantieri, and George J. Pasquerello. *Principles of Prolotherapy.* American Academy of Musculoskeletal Medicine, 2008.

K. Dean Reeves. "Sweet Relief." *Biomechanics*, 2004.

SPINE

Manuel Cusl, et al. "The Use of Prolotherapy in the Sacro-iliac Joint." *British Journal of Sports Medicine,* 2008.

Simon Dagenais, et al. "Evidence-informed Management of Chronic Low Back Pain with Prolotherapy." *Spine Journal,* 2008.

Simon Dagenais, et al. "Prolotherapy Injections for Chronic Low-back Pain." *Cochrane Database System Review,* 2007.

Sunny R. Kim, et al. "Critical Review of Prolotherapy for Osteoarthritis, Low Back Pain, and other Musculoskeletal Conditions." *Physiatric Perspective of Prolotherapy,* 2004.

Harold A. Wilkinson. "Injection therapy for Enthesopathies Causing Axial Spine Pain and 'The Failed Back Syndrome': A Single Blinded, Randomized and Cross-over Study." *Pain Physician,* 2005.

LOWER LEG

Norman J. Maxwell. "Sonographically Guided Intratendinous Injection of Hyperosmolar Dextrose to Treat Chronic Tendinosis of the Achilles Tendon: A Pilot Study." *Musculoskeletal Imaging,* 2007.

Mikel Sanchez, et al. "Comparison of Surgically Repaired Achilles Tendon Tears Using Platelet-rich Fibrin Matrices." *American Journal of Sports Medicine,* 2007.

Michael J. Yelland, et al. "Prolotherapy Injections and Eccentric Loading Exercises for Painful Achilles Tendinosis: A Randomised Trial." *British Journal of Sports Medicine,* 2011.

PELVIS

Gaston A. Topol, et al. "Efficacy of Dextrose Prolotherapy in Elite Male Kicking-sport Athletes with Chronic Groin Pain." *American Academy of Physical Medicine and Rehabilitation,* 2005.

KNEE

H. Alfredson and L. Ohberg. "Neovascularization in Chronic Painful Patellar Tendinosis: Promising Results after Sclerosing Neovessels Outside the Tendon Challenge the Need for Surgery." *Knee Surgery, Sports Traumatology, Arthroscopy,* 2005.

Richard Dumais, et al. "Effect of Regenerative Injection Therapy on Function and Pain in Patients with Knee Osteoarthritis: A Randomized Crossover Study." *Pain Medicine.* 2012.

K.T. Jensen, et al. "Early Inflammatory Response of Knee Ligaments to Prolotherapy in a Rat Model." *Journal of Orthopaedic Research,* 2009.

S.A. Kim, et al. "The Effects of Hyperosmolar Dextrose and Autologous Serum Injection in the Experimental Articular Defect of Rabbit." *The Journal of the Korean Academy of Rehabilitation Medicine,* 2002.

C. Pascual-Garrido, et al. "Treatment of Chronic Patellar Tendinopathy with Autologous Bone Marrow Stem Cells: A Five-year Follow-up." *Stem Cells International,* 2012.

David Rabago, et al. "Dextrose Prolotherapy for Knee Osteoarthritis: A Randomized Controlled Trial." *Annals of Family Medicine,* 2013.

David Rabago, et al. "Dextrose Prolotherapy for Knee Osteoarthritis: Results of a Randomized Controlled Trial." *Osteoarthritis and Cartilage.* 2011.

David Rabago, et al. "Hypertonic Dextrose Injections (Prolotherapy) for Knee Osteoarthritis: Results of a Single-arm Uncontrolled Study One-year Follow-up." *The Journal of Alternative and Complementary Medicine.* 2012.

K. Dean Reeves and Khatab Hassanein. "Randomized Prospective Double-blind Placebo-controlled Study of Dextrose Prolotherapy for Knee Osteoarthritis with or Without ACL Laxity." *Alternative Therapies,* 2000.

Gaston Andres Topol. "Arthroscopically Monitored Effects of Prolotherapy in Knee Osteoarthritis: Pilot Data." *UW Hackett-Hemwall Prolotherapy Research Symposium,* October 20, 2010.

Gaston Andres Topol, et al. "Hyperosmolar Dextrose Injection for Recalcitrant Osgood-Schlatter Disease." *Pediatrics,* 2011.

HEAD AND NECK

Roy V. Hakala. "Prolotherapy (Proliferation Therapy) in the Treatment of TMD." *The Journal of Craniomandibular Practice,* 2005.

R. Allan Hooper, et al. "Case Series on Chronic Whiplash Related Neck Pain Treated with Intraarticular Zygapophysial Joint Regeneration Injection Therapy." *Pain Physician,* 2007.

HAND AND ARM

Thomas M. Best, et al. "A Systematic Review of Four Injection Therapies for Lateral Epicondylosis: Prolotherapy, Polidocanol, Whole Blood and Platelet-rich Plasma." *British Journal of Sports Medicine,* 2009.

David Rabago. "David Rabago's Team Takes a Rigorous Look at Prolotherapy for Tennis Elbow." Fammed.wisc.edu. January 2012. Website: http://www.fammed.wisc.edu/our-department/newsletter/winter-2011/prolotherapy-tennis-elbow.

K. Dean Reeves and Khatab Hassanein. "Randomized, Prospective, Placebo-controlled Double-blind Study of Dextrose Prolotherapy for Osteoarthritic Thumb and Finger (DIP, PIP, and Trapeziometacarpal) Joints: Evidence of Clinical Efficacy." *Journal of Alternative and Complementary Medicine,* 2000.

Michael Scarpone, et al. "The Efficacy of Prolotherapy for Lateral Epicondylosis: A Pilot Study." *Clinical Journal of Sports Medicine,* 2008.

FOOT AND ANKLE

M.B. Ryan, et al. "Sonographically Guided Intratendinous Injections of Hyperosmolar Dextrose/Lidocaine: A Pilot Study for the Treatment of Plantar Fasciitis." *British Journal of Sports Medicine,* 2009.

ON SUPERFICIAL PERINEURAL INJECTIONS AND BIOPUNCTURE

S.D. Brain and P.K. Moore, eds. *Pain and Neurogenic Inflammation.* Birkhäuser 1999.

M.J. Caterina, et al. "The Capsaicin Receptor: A Heat-activated Ion Channel in the Pain Pathway." *Nature,* 1997.

Pierangelo Geppetti and Peter Holzer, eds. *Neurogenic Inflammation,* CRC Press, 1996.

Gabor Jancso, ed. *Neurogenic Inflammation in Health and Disease,* Vol. 8. Elsevier Science, 2009.

Jan Kersschot. *The Clinical Guide to Biopuncture.* Inspiration Publishers, 2010.

L. Kruger, et al. "Peripheral Patterns of Calcitonin-gene-related Peptide General Somatic Sensory Innervation: Cutaneous and Deep Terminations." *The Journal of Comparative Neurology,* 1989.

Annika B. Malmberg and Keith R. Bley, eds. *Turning up the Heat on Pain: TRPV1 Receptors in Pain and Inflammation.* Springer, 2005.

Sidney Ochs. *A History of Nerve Functions.* Cambridge University Press, 2004.

Douglas Zochodne. *Neurobiology of Peripheral Nerve Regeneration.* Cambridge University Press, 2008.

ON PLATELET-RICH PLASMA

David Crane and Peter A.M. Everts. "Platelet-rich Plasma (PRP) Matrix Grafts." *Practical Pain Management,* 2008.

H. El-Sharkawy, et al. "Platelet-rich Plasma: Growth Factors and Pro- and Anti-inflammatory Properties." *Journal of Periodontology,* 2007.

M. Ferrari, et al. "A New Technique for Hemodilution, Preparation of Autologous Platelet-rich Plasma and Intraoperative Blood Salvage in Cardiac Surgery." *International Journal of Artificial Organs,* 1987.

Illaria Giusti, et al. "Identification of an Optimal Concentration of Platelet Gel for Promoting Angiogenesis in Human Endothelial Cells." *Transfusion*, 2009.

Jason W. Hammond, et al. "Use of Autologous Platelet-rich Plasma to Treat Muscle Strain Injuries." *American Journal of Sports Medicine*, 2009.

Douglas W. Jackson, et al. "Accuracy of Needle Placement into the Intra Articular Space of the Knee." *Journal of Bone and Joint Surgery*, 2002.

D.R. Knighton, et al. "Classification and Treatment of Non-healing Wounds: Successful Treatment with Autologous Platelet-derived Wound Healing Factors (PDWHF)." *Annals of Surgery*, 1986.

A. Mishra and T. Pavelko. "Treatment of Chronic Elbow Tendinosis with Buffered Platelet-rich Plasma." *American Journal of Sports Medicine*, 2006.

Scott A. Rodeo, et al. "Platelet-Rich Plasma: From Basic Science to Clinical Applications." *American Journal of Sports Medicine*, 2009.

Steven Sampson. "Platelet Rich Plasma Injection Grafts for Musculoskeletal Injuries: A Review." *Current Reviews in Musculoskeletal Medicine*, 2008.

Michael A. Scarpone. "Chronic Medial Collateral High-grade Tear: Treatment with Autologous Platelet Concentrate Injection with Ultrasound Guidance: A Case Report." *HarvestTech.com*, 2007.

Michael A. Scarpone. "Non-Surgical Repair of High Grade Achilles Tendon Tear by Autologous Platelet Graft Placement: A Case Report." *HarvestTech.com*, 2007.

Allan Schwartz. "A Promising Treatment for Athletes, in Blood." *NYTimes.com*, February 16, 2009.

P. Volpi, et al. "Treatment of Chronic Patellar Tendinosis with Buffered Platelet-rich Plasma: A Preliminary Study." *Medicina Dello Sport*, 2007.

ON ADULT AUTOLOGOUS STEM CELL INJECTIONS

OVERVIEW

Todd Ackerman."Perry Brings His Stem-cell Cause to Houston." *Chron.com,* October 30, 2012. Website: http://www.chron.com/news/houston-texas/houston/article/Perry-brings-Texas-stem-cell-cause-to-Houston-3985899.php.

Donna Alderman, et al. "Stem Cell Prolotherapy in Regenerative Medicine: Background, Theory and Protocols." *Journal of Prolotherapy,* 2011.

Christopher J. Centeno, et al. "A Case Series of Percutaneous Treatment of Non-union Fractures with Autologous, Culture Expanded, Bone Marrow-derived, Mesenchymal Stem Cells and Platelet Lysate." *Journal of Bioengineering and Biomedical Science,* 2011.

Christopher J. Centeno and Stephen J. Faulkner. "The Use of Mesenchymal Stem Cells in Orthopedics" in *Stem Cells and Cancer Stem Cells, Volume 1.* Springer, 2012.

A. I. Chaplan. "Mesenchymal Stem Cells: The Past, the Present, the Future." *Cartilage,* 2010.

A. Dicker, et al. "Functional Studies of Mesenchymal Stem Cells Derived from Adult Human Adipose Tissue." *Experimental Cell Research,* 2005.

Christian Hendrich, et al. "Safety of Autologous Bone Marrow Aspiration Concentrate Transplantation: Initial Experiences in 101 Patients." *Orthopedic Reviews,* 2009.

Letter from Ellen F. Lazarus, Director, Division of Human Tissues, Department of Health and Human Services, Food and Drug Administration, to Mitchell S. Fuerst. Website: http://box.com/s/v8du7czi944s3xlblr5g.

H. Nejadnik, et al. "Autologous Bone Marrow Derived Mesenchymal Stem Cells Versus Autologous Chondrocyte Implantation: An Observational Cohort Study." *American Journal of Sports Medicine,* 2010.

P. A. Zuk, et al. "Human Adipose Tissue Is a Source of Multipotent Stem Cells." *Molecular Biology of the Cell,* 2002.

BONE

D. Dallari, et al. "In Vivo Study on the Healing of Bone Defects Treated with Bone Marrow Stromal Cells, Platelet-rich Plasma, and Freeze-dried Bone Allografts, Alone and in Combination." *Journal of Orthopaedic Research,* 2006.

J. Gessman, et al. "Regenerate Augmentation with Bone Marrow Concentrate after Traumatic Bone Loss," *Orthopedic Reviews,* 2012.

Philippe Hernigou, et al. "Percutaneous Autologous Bone-marrow Grafting for Nonunions. Surgical Technique." *Journal of Bone and Joint Surgery,* American Volume, 2006.

Mustafa Romih, et al. "The Vertebral Interbody Grafting Site's Low Concentration in Osteogenic Progenitors Can Greatly Benefit from Addition of Iliac Crest Bone Marrow." *European Spine Journal,* 2005.

PELVIS

Kevin J. Campbell, et al. "Treatment of a Hip Capsular Injury in a Professional Soccer Player with Platelet-rich Plasma and Bone Marrow Aspirate Concentrate Therapy." *Knee Surgery, Sports Traumatology, Arthroscopy,* 2012.

Christopher J. Centeno, et al. "Partial Regeneration of the Human Hip via Autologous Bone Marrow Nucleated Cell Transfer: A Case Study." *Pain Physician,* 2006.

V. Gangii, et al. "Stem Cell Therapy for Osteonecrosis of the Femoral Head." *Expert Opinion on Biological Therapy,* 2005.

Philippe Hernigou, et al. "Decrease in the Mesenchymal Stem-cell Pool in the Proximal Femur in Corticosteroid-induced Osteonecrosis." *Journal of Bone and Joint Surgery, British Volume,* 1999.

Philippe Hernigou and Francoise Beaujean. "Treatment of Osteonecrosis with Autologous Bone Marrow Grafting." *Clinical Orthopedics and Related Research,* 2002.

R. Kuroda, et al. "Treatment of a Full Thickness Articular Cartilage Defect in the Femoral Condyle of an Athlete with Autologous Bone Marrow Stromal Cells." *Osteoarthritis and Cartilage,* 2007.

KNEE

Christopher J. Centeno, et al. "Increased Knee Cartilage Volume in Degenerative Joint Disease Using Percutaneously Implanted, Autologous Mesenchymal Stem Cells," *Pain Physician,* 2008.

Lee Yee Han Dave, et al. "Mesenchymal Stem Cell Therapy in the Sports Knee: Where Are We in 2011?" *Sports Health,* 2012.

S. Wakitani, et al. "Autologous Bone Marrow Stromal Cell Transplantation for Repair of Full Thickness Articular Cartilage Defects in Human Patellae: Two Case Reports," *Cell Transplantation,* 2004.

S. Wakitani, et al. "Human Autologous Culture Expanded Bone Marrow Mesenchymal Cell Transplantation for Repair of Cartilage Defects in Osteoarthritic Knees," *Osteoarthritis and Cartilage,* 2002.

S. Wakitani, et al. "Repair of Articular Cartilage Defects in the Patello-femoral Joint with Autologous Bone Marrow Mesenchymal Cell Transplantation: Three Case Reports Involving Nine Defects in Five Knees," *Journal of Tissue Engineering and Regenerative Medicine,* 2007.

FOOT AND ANKLE

N. A. Smyth, et al. "Establishing Proof of Concept: Platelet-rich Plasma and Bone Marrow Aspirate Concentrate May Improve Cartilage Repair Following Surgical Treatment for Osteochondral Lesions of the Talus." *World Journal of Orthopedics,* 2012.

CARTILAGE

L. A. Fortier, et al. "Concentrated Bone Marrow Aspirate Improves Full-thickness Cartilage Repair Compared with Microfracture in the Equine Model." *Journal of Bone and Joint Surgery, American Volume,* 2010.

S. Giannini, et al. "One-step Bone Marrow-derived Cell Transplantation in Talar Osteochondral Lesions," *Clinical Orthopaedics and Related Research,* 2009.

A. M. Haleem, et al. "The Clinical Use of Human Culture-expanded Autologous Bone Marrow Mesenchymal Stem Cells Transplanted on Platelet-rich Fibrin Glue in the Treatment of Articular Cartilage Defects: A Pilot Study and Preliminary Results." *Cartilage,* 2010.

A.P. Hollander, et al. "Stem Cells and Cartilage Development: Complexities of a Simple Tissue." *Stem Cells,* 2010.

J. I. Huang, et al. "Chondrogenic Potential of Progenitor Cells Derived from Human Bone Marrow: A Patient-matched Comparison." *Journal of Orthopedic Research,* 2005.

J. H. Hui, et al. "Treatment of Chondral Lesions in Advanced Osteochondritis Dissecanas: A Comparative Study of the Efficacy of Chondrocytes, Mesenchymal Stem Cells, Periosteal Graft and Mosaicplasty (Osteochondral Autograft) in Animal Models," *Journal of Orthopaedics,* 2004.

E. B. Hunziker and L. C. Rosenberg. "Repair of Partial-thickness Defects in Articular Cartilage: Cell Recruitment from the Synovial Membrane." *Journal of Bone and Joint Surgery, American Volume,* 1996.

H. Koga, et al. "Mesenchymal Stem Cell Based Therapy for Cartilage Repair: A Review." *Knee Surgery, Sports Traumatology, Arthroscopy,* 2009.

K. B. L. Lee, et al. "Injectable Mesenchymal Stem Cell Therapy for Large Cartilage Defects: A Porcine Model." *Stem Cells,* 2007.

K. Y. Saw, et al. "Articular Cartilage Regeneration with Autologous Marrow Aspirate and Hyaluronic Acid: An Experimental Study in a Goat Model," *Arthroscopy,* 2009.

K. Y. Saw, et al. "Articular Cartilage Regeneration with Autologous Peripheral Blood Progenitor Cells and Hyaluronic Acid after Arthroscopic Subchondral Drilling: A Report of Five Cases with Histology." *Arthroscopy,* 2011.

F. Veronesi,' et al. "Clinical Use of Bone Marrow, Bone Marrow Concentrate, and Expanded Bone Marrow Mesenchymal Stem Cells in Cartilage Disease." *Stem Cells and Development,* 2013.

OSTEOARTHRITIS

F.H. Chen and R.S. Tuan. "Mesenchymal Stem Cells in Arthritic Diseases," *Arthritis Research and Therapy,* 2008.

M.B. Goldring and S.R. Goldring. "Articular Cartilage and Subchondral Bone in the Pathogenesis of osteoarthritis." *Annals of the New York Academy of Sciences,* 2010.

Pawan K. Gupta, et al. "Mesenchymal Stem Cells for Cartilage Repair in Osteoarthritis." *Stem Cell Research and Therapy,* 2012.

S. Koelling and N. Miosge. "Stem Cell Therapy for Cartilage Regeneration in Osteoarthritis." *Expert Opinion on Biological Therapy,* 2009.

Jasvinder A. Singh. "Stem Cells and Other Innovative Intra-articular Therapies for Osteoarthritis: What Does the Future Hold?" *BMC Medicine,* 2012.

OTHER DISORDERS

Augusto Brazzini, et al. "Intraarterial Autologous Implantation of Adult Stem Cells for Patients with Parkinson's Disease." *Journal of Vascular and Interventional Radiology,* 2010.

Masaaki Kitada and Mari Dezawa. "Parkinson's Disease and Mesenchymal Stem Cells: Potential for Cell-based Therapy." *Parkinson's Disease,* 2011.

G. Mancardi and R Saccardi. "Autologous Hemaetopoietic Stem-cell Transplantation in Multiple Sclerosis." *Lancet Neurology,* 2008.

Kathleen Raven. "First US Stem Cell Trial for Autistic Children Launches Today." *Spoonful of Medicine,* August 21, 2012. Website: http://blogs.nature.com/spoonful/2012/08/first-us-stem-cell-trial-for-autistic-children-launches-today.html.

ACKNOWLEDGEMENTS

Regenerative Healing for Life has taken years to travel the journey from idea to a finished book. Many people have helped along the way. I trust I will remember most of them by name, but want to begin by thanking those I may inadvertently forget, as well as those whose privacy I am respecting by not mentioning them by name. Among these are the more than 10,000 patients who have trusted me with their new-healing-paradigm health care for more than a decade. I have learned a lesson from each of you that has helped me to become a better doctor. I particularly want to thank those patients willing to be interviewed for this book. Your contribution of your stories has been very valuable, both in illustrating what these treatments can do and in making these new methods easier for readers to understand.

Many other physicians have helped me come to my understanding of the new healing paradigm and how it can work to help patients with musculoskeletal injuries. I particularly want to thank Jeffrey Patterson, D.O., one of the "fathers" of modern-day prolotherapy and an invaluable mentor to me. I also thank my first clinical prolotherapy mentors, Jean Paul Ouellette, M.D., and Carl Osborn, D.O. I learned the foundations of the methods I use on all my prolotherapy patients from these three amazing doctors. They are all part of the Hackett Hemwall Foundation (HHF). The HHF is a premier organization that conducts research and teaches prolotherapy techniques to doctors and residents from a score of countries. It is housed at the University of Wisconsin School of Medicine, with Dr. Patterson as its caretaker. I have been part of numerous HHF trips to Honduras to help care for the under-served population of that country while teaching prolotherapy to other doctors. I have the honor of serving on the HHF board and have the greatest respect for all the members of the organiza-tion. Special thanks to all my friends in the HHF, especially David Rabago, M.D., my research mentor, and Andrew Kochan, M.D., an immeasurably talented prolotherapist and teacher of physicians, as well as my personal prolotherapist, dive buddy, and friend.

I have proudly worked with a variety of other organizations that have helped me come to a better understanding of the new paradigm. To my friends on the board of the American Associ-ation of Orthopaedic Medicine (AAOM), such as Drs. Bjorn Eek, Mayo Friedlis, and Tommy Bond, among several others, I am honored to serve and teach our members with your help to bring these new-paradigm healing methods to all of our patients. I was also the director of their research oversight committee, su-pervising the yearly budget for overseas research on RIT for the hip and knee, and the landmark randomized control trial on Os-good-Schlatter Disease published in the journal *Pediatrics*. I run a diagnostic ultrasound course for their annual pre-conference workshop, and have often lectured on prolotherapy topics. I have also taught diagnostic ultrasound, prolotherapy, and PRP at their annual summer workshop in Denver.

Thanks to the American Medical Society for Sports Medicine (AMSSM) for the opportunity to present several well-received prolotherapy workshops at their annual conference. I have also helped teach basic and advanced diagnostic ultrasound at their annual pre-conference. I am a founding board member of the International Cellular Medicine Society (ICMS) and have served on their PRP committee. I am working with them to help create a standard of care for the use of PRP, as well as to establish a registry of patients who have had the procedure.

I offer a special thanks to Colonel Francis O'Connor, M.D., who gave me the opportunity to present prolotherapy as a viable sports medicine treatment option first to the Marine Corps Marathon Symposium, and then, when he was serving on the board, to the AMSSM membership.

I also want to thank my good friend Colonel Sean Mulvaney, M.D., who has helped push cellular medicine and the use of high-resolution diagnostic ultrasound to the forefront (aka, point of the spear) of military medicine. You are a talented treasure to the men and women you serve. I understand your strong desire to continue to serve with, and for the people who make up your community. I'm sure I am in a long line of employers when I say that you will always have a place to continue your career when you are finished serving your country. I am honored to call both of these dedicated military men friends, and I want to publicly thank them both for their years of service to our country. We are forever in your debt.

There have been a number of well-known doctors who have also supported me in my work. I give particular thanks to Philadelphia orthopedic surgeon Arthur R. Bartolozzi, M.D., who has worked as the team physician for the Philadelphia Eagles and the Philadelphia Flyers. Special thanks also to Victor R. Kalman, D.O., of the Morgan Kalman Clinic in Wilmington, Delaware. He has cared for many sports greats, including baseball's Curt Schilling. Special appreciation also goes to Larry Nassar, D.O., a professor and team physician at Michigan State University who works with many Olympic athletes. I also thank Joseph Torg, M.D., John Kelly IV, M.D., and the deceased John Gregg, M.D., who accepted a young, non-operative sports medicine doctor into their orthopedic surgery club, Philadelphia Orthopedic Society for Sports Medicine (POSSM), long before the medical community of Philadelphia knew what to make of these new techniques. These legends of sports medicine didn't always see or believe in the value of prolotherapy to the sports medicine patient, but they did give the treatment a chance to be presented at annual research meetings. We even won third prize one year with our tennis elbow study.

I would like to especially thank Christopher J. Centeno, M.D., of Regenexx for his help with the stem cell section of the book. I acknowledge his tireless efforts to advance the technology of stem cells in interventional orthopedic medicine, and his willingness to challenge the FDA rulings so that physicians in the United States may one day be able to offer the most advanced stem cell techniques to patients. I also thank the other principals of Regenexx, John Schultz, M.D., Ronald Hanson, M.D., and Carl Measer, M.B.A., for cordially accepting me into the Regenexx family network. With you, I look forward to many years of successful progress in the new specialty of Interventional Orthopedic Medicine.

It is with gratitude that I acknowledge Tom Clark, D.C., my friend and mentor in diagnostic ultrasound. You have taken me from a poseur to an expert. I owe you my ability to see into my patients' bodies with a new set of eyes. I look forward to one day helping you teach diagnostic ultrasound to physicians in far-away lands. I would like to thank my friends who have been long-standing teachers in Tom Clark's Musculoskeletal Ultrasound (MSKUS) company, Paul Tortland, D.O., Albert Kozar, D.O., and Robert Monaco, M.D. I have spent many a weekend not only teaching others, but being taught by all of you. It's been a collective experience of *esprit de corps*. I have learned much and have enjoyed our friendship and continued efforts to drive this technology forward.

Special thanks also go to John Lyftogt, M.D., from New Zealand for his tireless work developing and teaching the perineural superficial injections (PSI) form of RIT.

I appreciate all of the experience I gained treating sports injuries when I acted as Chief Medical Officer for the Keystone State Games, for the Pennsylvania Senior Games, and for the Philadelphia Triathlon. I learned much as a team physician for the one-hundredth running of the Boston Marathon, for the McDonald's Ladies Professional Golf Association for the Classic Professional Golfers Association, for the U.S. Figure Skating Championships, for the U.S. Olympic Committee Training Center, and as a liaison team physician for the San Francisco Giants Baseball Team when they played in Philadelphia. I gained more knowledge working as a consulting team physician for the University of Delaware, where their team physician, Andrew Reisman, M.D., referred wonderful athletes to me and challenged me to use prolotherapy and platelet-rich plasma (PRP) to help his acutely injured athletes return to their teams as quickly as possible. I also worked at a number of high schools as a team physician for football, wrestling and hockey.

While I was gaining all of this experience and beginning to conquer all of the challenges that have marked my career in sports medicine, my wife, Eileen, was a constant source of emotional support while also doing a wonderful job of raising our three daughters. The young women they have become are a tribute to her talents as their mother. I appreciate all the love and support these women give me on a daily basis. I apologize to each of them for not being there so many nights and weekends when I was serving as a team physician or a board member, or was lecturing to a group of physicians somewhere on the planet. My lovely and talented daughter Kelly is on her way to becoming a physician's assistant. I am so proud of her and trust her career in medicine will be as rewarding for her as mine has been for me. I hope she will enthusiastically get up each morning as I do, looking forward to the challenges my patients will present to me. I am equally as proud of our incredibly artistic daughter Bridget whose talents are taking her to an exciting new direction in her life. She has grown into an amazingly beautiful woman inside and out. And to my youngest, Clare, I thank you for the carefree escape from everyday life through the eyes of you, my youngest, truly wonderful child.

I thank both my family and Eileen's Harkins family for their unwavering support. Special thanks to my father and mother, Edward and Patricia Shiple, who instilled their children with the ability to do our best in all we do and to make our dreams a reality once we put our minds to it.

I thank my office staff at the Center for Sports Medicine for making sure things go smoothly when I'm seeing patients and doing procedures. Special thanks to Lindsey DeProspero, Julia Barnett, Patty Dougherty, and Jacylyn Adams.

Special thanks to my co-author, Marlise Wind, for seeing the potential for a book that would interest the general public in regenerative healing. It took her close to a decade of constantly reminding me that I needed to find time to talk with her and write to make this dream a reality.

I thank you for buying *Regenerative Healing for Life* and for being open to the concept of a new paradigm for healing injuries and pain without surgery. May the ideas in this book help you to achieve and maintain the best possible health.

Brian J. Shiple, D.O.
July 2013

I thank Dr. Brian Shiple for his deeply compassionate care for all of his patients, and for his courage in pursuing the remarkable, cutting-edge medicine he practices. It has kept me moving with as little surgery or bionic parts as possible. Special thanks to my husband, Thomas Wind, D.O., another dedicated physician who truly cares for his patients' welfare. Understanding his schedule and the demands of his calling made it easier for me to comprehend and work around Dr. Shiple's schedule. And Tom was often there to explain the meaning of medical terms at the sometimes late hours when I was working. Special thanks also to our daughter Kyla, a beautiful young woman inside and out, and a talented, hardworking artist, organizer, and communicator. Your warm, confident, nurturing, questioning nature is always an inspiration. Thanks to my offices away from home, where, in the absence of stone and mortar bookstores, I can think, write, and focus only on my work: Panera, Starbucks, and the other free Wi-Fi havens where artists can gather.

My thanks to our extremely competent editor, Stephany Evans, of Fine Print Literary Agency and Lincoln Square Books; to Stephanie Gunning, our knowledgeable, always enthusiastic production manager; and to Peter Rubie, our fastidious copyeditor. An appreciative acknowledgement also goes to P.M.H. Atwater, a dear, longtime friend who introduced me to Stephany Evans, who had been her agent and is now mine. My appreciation also goes to Sarah Rachel Evans, my meticulous, tenacious, affable research and technology assistant, who was always willing to be there to ensure my conversations with Dr. Shiple were properly recorded and summarized, sometimes late into the evening. She used all of her Vassar training to be sure the research, recommended reading list, grammar, commas, and most importantly, endnotes in the book were up to par. Thanks also to Dorothy (Dot) Butscher, my friend and office assistant, who was always there with encouragement and organization. Thanks also to others who cheered me on in writing: especially the late Dorothy (Dorrie) Sellers, Georgianne James, Heidi Jacob, Charles Abramovic and Robert Abramovic, Peter and Fran Neall, Lisa Sachs, Jean Thorne, Karen Norris, and Jean and Jack Sargent. Special thanks to Richard Schwartzman, D.O., a most knowledgeable physician and human being who has greatly improved my sense of humor and taught me to look for truth and beauty in every moment of life.

I thank Gus Yoo, who did an excellent job of designing the book. Thanks also to June Clark for her help in spreading the word about the book to as many people as possible. My sincere thanks goes to all the people who told me their amazing stories of healing. You are each an inspiration to me and will be to many other people.

May this book bring this cutting-edge, often miraculous medicine into the mainstream where it can help so many others who are suffering needlessly.

Marlise Wind

July 2013

END NOTES

INTRODUCTION

1. C. Everett Koop, "Appendix C: Letter from C. Everett Koop," in *Healing Back and Joint Injuries: A Proven Approach to Ending Chronic Pain and Avoiding Unnecessary Surgery* by Joseph Valdez (Austin, TX.: Greenleaf Book Group Press, 2009): p. 232.

2. Allan Schwartz, "A Promising Treatment for Athletes, in Blood," NYTimes.com (posted February 16, 2009, accessed June 21, 2009). Website: http://www.nytimes.com/2009/02/17/sports/17blood.html.

3. American Academy of Orthopaedic Surgeons, "Orthopaedic Fast Facts," Orthoinfo.AAOS.org (posted May 1, 2009, accessed August 16, 2012). Website: http://orthoinfo.aaos.org/topic.cfm?topic=A00130#A00130_R1_anchor.

4. National Center for Chronic Disease Prevention and Health Promotion, Division of Population Health, "Arthritis Related Statistics,"CDC.gov (posted August 1, 2011, accessed August 16, 2012). Centers for Disease Control and Prevention
Website: http://www.cdc.gov/arthritis/data_statistics/arthritis_related_stats.htm.

5. American Academy of Orthopaedic Surgeons, "Orthopaedic Fast Facts."

6. Ibid.

7. N. Mahomed, et al., "The Self-administered Patient Satisfaction Scale for Primary Hip and Knee Arthroplasty," *Arthritis*, vol. 2011, Article ID 591253 (2011): 6 pages.

8. Michael J. Yelland, et al., "Prolotherapy Injections and Eccentric Loading Exercises for Painful Achilles Tendinosis: A Randomised Trial," *British Journal of Sports Medicine*, vol. 45, no. 5 (2011): pp. 421–8.

CHAPTER TWO

1. Thomas H. Ravin, Mark S. Cantieri, and George J. Pasquerello, *Principles of Prolotherapy.* Denver, CO.: (American Academy of Musculoskeletal Medicine, 2008).

2. Joseph A. DiMasi, et al., "The Price of Innovation: New Estimates of Drug Development Costs," *Journal of Health Economics*, vol. 22 (2003): pp. 151–85.

3. Allan F. Shaughnessey and Jay Siwek, "Editorials: Introducing POEMs," *American Family Physician*, vol. 67, no. 6 (March 2003): pp. 1196–9.

4. Centre for Evidence-based Medicine, "Levels of Evidence," CEBM.net (posted March 2009, accessed November 9, 2012). Website: http://www.cebm.net/index.aspx?o=1025.

CHAPTER THREE

1. American Academy of Orthopaedic Surgeons, "Orthopaedic Fast Facts," Orthoinfo.AAOS.org (posted May 1, 2009, accessed August 16, 2012). Website: http://orthoinfo.aaos.org/topic.cfm?topic=A00130#A00130_R1_anchor.

2. National Center for Injury Prevention and Control, "Injury: The Leading Cause of Death Among Persons 1–44," CDC.gov (accessed June 9, 2011). Centers for Disease Control and Prevention Website: http://www.cdc.gov/injury/overview/leading_cod.html.

3. Ibid.

4. National Center for Injury Control and Prevention, "Table 2: Unintentional Injury Deaths, All Ages, All Races/Ethnicities, Both Sexes—United States, 2005," *CDC Injury Research Agenda, 2009–2018* (Atlanta, GA.: US Department of Health and Human Services, Centers for Disease Control and Prevention, 2009): p. 10.

5. Department of Health and Human Services, *CDC Injury Research Agenda* (Atlanta, GA.: Centers for Disease Prevention and Control, National Center for Injury Prevention and Control, 2002): p. 85.

6. Ibid.

7. Ibid.

8. Y. J. Cheng, et al., "Prevalence of Doctor-diagnosed Arthritis and Arthritis-attributable Activity Limitation—United States, 2007–2009," *Morbidity and Mortality Weekly Report*, vol. 59, no. 39 (October 8, 2010): pp. 1261–5. Centers for Disease Control and Prevention Website: http://www.cdc.gov/mmwr/preview/mmwrhtml/mm5939a1.htm.

9. Ibid.

10. David C. Reid M.D., *Sports Injury Assessment and Rehabilitation* (Philadelphia, PA.: Churchill Livingstone, 1991).

11. I first heard about the concept of dynamic stabilization from James A. Porterfield. His article "Dynamic Stabilization of the Trunk" appeared in the March/April 1985 issue of *The Journal of Orthopedic and Sports Physical Therapy*, pp. 271–7. I have used his work to posit dynamic stabilization failure.

12. Reid.

13. S.A. Itay, et al., "Clinical and Functional Status Following Lateral Ankle Sprains," *Orthopaedic Review*, vol.11, no. 5 (1982): pp. 73–6.

14. Scott W. Atlas, M.D., "Let's Be Honest—Medicare Is Insolvent and Doctors Soon Won't Accept It," *Forbes Online* (posted December 18, 2012, accessed January 12, 2013). Website: www.forbes.com/sites/scottatlas/2012/12/18/lets-be-honest-medicare-is-insolvent-and-doctors-soon-wont-accept-it/

15. American Association of Hip and Knee Surgeons, "Frequently Asked Questions," AAHKS.org (posted October 10, 2008, accessed October 27, 2012). Website: http://www.aahks.org/patients/documentary/inside_look.asp.

16. Ibid.

17. R. Gandhi, et al., "Predicting Patient Dissatisfaction Following Joint Replacement Surgery," *Journal of Rheumatology*, vol. 35, no. 12 (December 2008): pp. 2415–8.

18. American Academy of Orthopaedic Surgeons, "Baseball Injury Prevention," Orthoinfo.AAOS.org (posted June 2011, accessed November 14, 2012). Website: http://orthoinfo.aaos.org/topic.cfm?topic=A00185.

CHAPTER FOUR

1. Melissa Conrad Stöppler, "Treating a Sprained Ankle," Emedicinehealth.com (posted July 2, 2008, accessed July 17, 2012). Website: http://www.emedicinehealth.com/ankle_sprain/article_em.htm.

2. American Medical Society for Sports Medicine brochure, *The Sports Medicine Specialist* (Overland Park, KS., 2002).

3. M.A. Slatyer, M.J. Hensley, and R. Lopert, "A Randomized Controlled Trial of Piroxicam in the Management of Acute Ankle Sprain in Australian Regular Army Recruits: The Kapooka Ankle Sprain Study," *American Journal of Sports Medicine*, vol. 25, no. 4 (July–August 1997): pp. 544–53.

4. Ibid.

5. These are the average statistics most commonly cited, although the numbers of deaths vary widely depending on the source of the story.

6. Emil Loldrup Fosbøl, et al., "Cause-specific Cardiovascular Risk Associated with Nonsteroidal Anti-inflammatory Drugs among Healthy Individuals," *Circulation: Cardiovascular Quality and Outcomes*, vol. 3 (July 2010): pp. 395–405.

7. J. F. Reynolds, et al., "Non-steroidal Anti-inflammatory Drugs Fail to Enhance Healing of Acute Hamstring Injuries Treated with Physiotherapy," *South African Medical Journal*, vol. 85 (1995): pp. 517–22.

8. M.R. Carmont, et al., "Simultaneous Bilateral Achilles Tendon Ruptures Associated with Statin Medication Despite Regular Rock Climbing Exercise," *Physical Therapy in Sport,* vol. 10, no. 4 (November 2009): pp. 150–2.

9. P. Otruba, et al., "Treatment with Statins and Peripheral Neuropathy: Results of 36-Months a Prospective Clinical and Neurophysiological Follow-up," *Neuro Endocrinology Letters*, vol. 32, no. 5 (2011): pp. 688–90.

10. Philippe Hernigou, et al., "Decrease in the Mesenchymal Stem-cell Pool in the Proximal Femur in Corticosteroid-induced Osteonecrosis," *Journal of Bone and Joint Surgery, British Volume*, vol. 81, no. 2 (March 1999): pp. 349–55.

11. Sally Arno, et al, "The Effect of Arthroscopic Partial Medial Meniscectomy on Tibiofemoral Stability," *American Journal of Sports Medicine*, vol. 41, no. 1 (January 2013): pp. 73-79.

12. Mark M. Mikhael, et al., "Failure of Metal-on-metal Total Hip Arthroplasty Mimicking Hip Infection: A Report of Two Cases," *American Journal of Bone and Joint Surgery*, vol. 91, no. 2 (February 2009): pp. 443–6.

CHAPTER FIVE

1. To read Dr. Still's story and the basic principles of osteopathy, consult Andrew Taylor Still, *The Philosophy and Mechanical Principles of Osteopathy* (Kansas City, MO.: Hudson-Kimberly Publishing Company, 1902).

2. To read Dr. Palmer's story and become familiar with the basic concepts of chiropractic medicine, consult Daniel David Palmer, *The Chiropractor's Adjuster* (Portland, OR.: Portland Printing House, 1910.)

3. This is a measure of clinical improvement described in the orthopedic literature as a standard goal.

4. "Historical Note," Janet G. Travell papers, University Archives, Special Collections Research Center, The George Washington University (accessed January 12, 2013). Website: http://www.gwu.edu/gelman/spec/ead/ms0704.xml#ref1697.

5. Janet G. Travell and David G. Simons, Travell and Simons' *Myofascial Pain and Dysfunction: The Trigger Point Manual, volume 1, second edition* (Philadelphia, PA.: Lippincott Williams & Wilkins, 1999): p. 52.

6. Jay P. Shah and Elizabeth A. Gilliams, "Uncovering the Biochemical Milieu of Myofascial Trigger Points Using in Vivo Microdialysis: An Application of Muscle Pain Concepts to Myofascial Pain Syndrome," *Journal of Bodywork and Movement Therapies*, no. 12 (October 2008): pp. 371–84.

7. S. Williams, et al., "Kinesio Taping in Treatment and Prevention of Sports

Injuries: A Meta-analysis of the Evidence for Its Effectiveness," *Journal of Orthopedic and Sports Physical Therapy,* vol. 42, no. 2 (February 2012): pp. 153–64.

8. Christopher McDougall, *Born to Run* (New York: Alfred A. Knopf, 2009).

CHAPTER SIX

1. This was named after Tommy John, the first professional pitcher whose career was prolonged by this reconstructive procedure.

2. Biloine W. Young, "Young Patients Getting Tommy John Surgery," RYOrtho.com (posted December 7, 2011, accessed August 20, 2012). Website: http://ryortho.com/extremities.php?news=1605_Young-Patients-Getting-Tommy-John-Surgery.

3. Michael Scarpone, et al., "The Efficacy of Prolotherapy for Lateral Epicondylosis: A Pilot Study," *Clinical Journal of Sports Medicine*, vol. 18, no. 3 (May 2008): pp. 248–54.

CHAPTER SEVEN

1. Janet G. Travell and David G. Simons, *Myofascial Pain and Dysfunction: The Trigger Point Manual, volume 2, second edition* (Philadelphia, PA.: Lippincott Williams & Wilkins, 1998).

2. Simon Dagenais, et al., "Intraligamentous Injections of Sclerosing Solutions (Prolotherapy) for Spinal Pain: A Critical Review of the Literature," *Spine Journal,* vol. 5 (2005): pp. 324.

3. R. Bellamy, "Compensation Neurosis: Financial Reward for Illness as Nocebo," *Clinical Orthopaedics and Related Research*, no. 336 (March 1997): pp. 94–106.

CHAPTER EIGHT

1. PSI began in New Zealand, and was first formally taught to physicians in 2006.

2. Juliana Maude Bue-Valleskey, et al., *Methods of Treating Neuropeptide Y-associated Conditions*. United States of America Patent EP0754464 A2. January 22, 1997.

3. Michael J. Yelland, et al., "Prolotherapy Injections and Eccentric Loading Exercises for Painful Achilles Tendinosis: A Randomised Trial," *British Journal of Sports Medicine*, vol. 45, no. 5 (2011): pp. 421–8.

4. This comes from data that John Lyftogt, M.D., presented at the Twenty-eighth Annual AAOM Conference in June 2011, which is extrapolated from statistics relating to the patients he has treated in his practice.

5. Robert Maigne, M.D., from France, did painstaking dissections of thirty-plus cadavers to elucidate the anatomy of the superficial nerves (cluneal plexus) of the low back. He wrote about his work in *Diagnosis and Treatment of Pain of Vertebral Origin, second edition* (London, U.K.: CRC Press, 2005). He believes at least 30 percent of patients with low back pain suffer from injury to these superficial nerves. He believes this is the most overlooked potential pain generator for low back pain, and I agree with his findings, as I have learned to pay attention to these pain generators in my low back pain patients.

6. Sample website: http://www/saferpills.org.

7. This comes from data that John Lyftogt, M.D., presents in his workshops. He has extrapolated this from his own statistics taken from the data he has collected from patients he has treated and followed in his practice in New Zealand.

8. For more information about Dr. Kersschot and biopuncture, consult Jan Kersschot, *The Clinical Guide to Biopuncture* (Aartselaar, Belgium: Inspiration Publishers, 2010).

9. I have found Traumeel and Lymphomyosot to have a similar effect compared to dextrose. Some specialists in regenerative medicine now are routinely adding Traumeel to their PRP injections for added anti-inflammatory relief. These medications offer another alternative to steroid injections or synthetic joint fluids. More research is needed to understand the role of these medications. A remedy like Traumeel is complex with fourteen ingredients, including Arnica Montana. Slowly, quality research on key ingredients in the Traumeel formulation has been entering mainstream

medicine. Arnica is probably the most commonly used homeopathic remedy in the world. Recently, two important plastic surgery randomized controlled studies tested Arnica and its effects on recovery from bruising and swelling after rhinoplasty. Patients who took Arnica instead of the standard steroids had a statistically significant quicker resolution of bruising.

10. S. Porozov, et al., "Inhibition of IL-1 Beta and TNF-alpha Secretion from Resting and Activated Human Immunocytes by the Homeopathic Medication Traumeel S," *Clinical and Developmental Immunology*, vol. 11, no. 2 (June 2004): pp. 143–9.

CHAPTER NINE

1. Allen H. Minor, M.D., and Lee Barnett, M.S., "Clinical Experience of Transfusions of Platelets Separated from Normal Blood," *Journal of the American Medical Association*, vol. 152, no. 13 (July 1953): pp. 1225–7.

2. M. Ferrari, et al., "A New Technique for Hemodilution, Preparation of Autologous Platelet-rich Plasma and Intraoperative Blood Salvage in Cardiac Surgery," *International Journal of Artificial Organs*, vol. 10, no. 1 (January 1987): pp. 47–50.

3. D.R. Knighton, et al., "Classification and Treatment of Non-healing Wounds: Successful Treatment with Autologous Platelet-derived Wound Healing Factors (PDWHF)," *Annals of Surgery*, vol. 204, no. 3 (September 1986): pp. 322–30.

4. A. Mishra and T. Pavelko, "Treatment of Chronic Elbow Tendinosis with Buffered Platelet-rich Plasma," *American Journal of Sports Medicine*, no. 34 (2006): pp. 1774–8.

5. Ibid.

6. Ibid.

7. For further information, refer to http://www.Regenexx.com.

8. Allan Schwartz, "A Promising Treatment for Athletes, in Blood," NYTimes. com (posted February 16, 2009, accessed June 21, 2009). Website: http://www.nytimes.com/2009/02/17/sports/17blood.html.

9. Allan Mishra, et al., "Treatment of Tendon and Muscle Using Platelet-rich Plasma," *Clinical Sports Medicine*, no. 28 (2009): pp. 113–25.

10. Illaria Giusti, et al., "Identification of an Optimal Concentration of Platelet Gel for Promoting Angiogenesis in Human Endothelial Cells," *Transfusion*, vol. 49, no. 4 (April 2009): pp. 771–8.

11. For an expanded discussion of how flawed and biased articles affect how doctors use PRP and other aspects of RIT, please see Chapter Fifteen.

12. Douglas W. Jackson, et al., "Accuracy of Needle Placement into the Intra Articular Space of the Knee," *Journal of Bone and Joint Surgery*, vol. 84, no. 9 (September 2002): pp. 1522–7.

13. There is anecdotal evidence from patients (and the author, as a patient) that this is the case.

CHAPTER TEN

1. For further information about worldwide developments in stem cell methods and technology, please refer to Chapter Fifteen.

2. Lee Yee Han Dave, et al., "Mesenchymal Stem Cell Therapy in the Sports Knee: Where Are We in 2011?" *Sports Health*, vol. 4, no. 3 (May 2012): pp. 252–7.

3. Letter from Ellen F. Lazarus, Director, Division of Human Tissues, Department of Health and Human Services, Food and Drug Administration, to Mitchell S. Fuerst, Esquire (posted November 2011, accessed November 19, 2012). Website: http://box.com/s/v8du7czi944s3xlblr5g.

4. Donna Alderman, et al., "Stem Cell Prolotherapy in Regenerative Medicine: Background, Theory and Protocols," *Journal of Prolotherapy*, vol. 3, no. 3 (August 2011): pp. 689–708.

5. R.S. Carpenter, et al., "Osteoblastic Differentiation of Human and Equine Adult Bone Marrow-derived Mesenchymal Stem Cells when BMP-2 or BMP-7 Homodimer Genetic Modification Is Compared to BMP-2/7 Heterodimer Genetic Modification in the Presence and Absence of Dexa-

methasone," *Journal of Orthopaedic Research*, vol. 28, no. 10 (2010): pp. 1330–7.

6. Philippe Hernigou and Francoise Beaujean, "Treatment of Osteonecrosis with Autologous Bone Marrow Grafting," *Clinical Orthopedics and Related Research*, vol. 405 (December 2002): pp. 14–23.

7. C.J. Centeno, et al., "A Case Series of Percutaneous Treatment of Nonunion Fractures with Autologous, Culture Expanded, Bone Marrow-derived, Mesenchymal Stem Cells and Platelet Lysate," *Journal of Bioengineering and Biomedical Science,* S2 (2011): p. 7. Website: http://www.omicsonline.org/2155-9538/2155-9538-S2-007.pdf.

8. C.J. Centeno, et al., "Increased Knee Cartilage Volume in Degenerative Joint Disease Using Percutaneously Implanted, Autologous Mesenchymal Stem Cells," *Pain Physician*, vol. 11, no. 3 (2008): pp. 343–53.

9. Christopher J. Centeno and Stephen J. Faulkner, "The Use of Mesenchymal Stem Cells in Orthopedics," *Stem Cells and Cancer Stem Cells, Volume 1,* edited by M.A. Hayat (New York: Springer, 2012): pp.173–9.

10. R.H. Demling and D.P. Orgill, "The Anticatabolic and Wound Healing Effects of the Testosterone Analog Oxandrolone after Severe Burn Injury," *Journal of Critical Care*, vol. 15, no. 1 (March 2000): pp. 12–17.

11. Mark Frankle and Joseph Borrelli, "The Effects of Testosterone Propionate and Methenolone Enanthate on the Healing of Humeral Osteotomies in the Wistar Rat," *Journal of Investigative Surgery*, vol. 3, no. 2 (1990): pp. 93–113.

12. Gaston Andres Topol, "Arthroscopically Monitored Effects of Prolotherapy in Knee Osteoarthritis: Pilot Data," UW Hackett-Hemwall Prolotherapy Research Symposium (Madison, WI.: University of Wisconsin School of Medicine and Public Health, October 20, 2010).

13. H. El-Sharkawy, et al., "Platelet-rich Plasma: Growth Factors and Pro- and Anti-inflammatory Properties," *Journal of Periodontology*, vol. 78, no. 4 (April 2007): pp. 661–9.

14. Allen Mask, "Duke Explores Stem Cell Treatment for Children with Cerebral Palsy," WRAL.com (posted May 12, 2011, accessed November 29, 2012). Website: http://www.wral.com/lifestyles/healthteam/story/9587943.

15. G. Mancardi and R. Saccardi, "Autologous Hemaetopoietic Stem-cell Transplantation in Multiple Sclerosis," *Lancet Neurology*, vol. 7, no. 7 (July 2008): pp. 626–36.

16. Masaaki Kitada and Mari Dezawa, "Parkinson's Disease and Mesenchymal Stem Cells: Potential for Cell-based Therapy," *Parkinson's Disease*, vol. 2012 (November 2011): p. 9.

17. Augusto Brazzini, et al., "Intraarterial Autologous Implantation of Adult Stem Cells for Patient's with Parkinson's Disease," *Journal of Vascular and Interventional Radiology*, vol. 21, no. 4 (April 2010): pp. 443–51.

18. "Autologous Stem Cell Therapy (ASCT) with Parkinson's Patients," Foundation for Alternative and Integrative Medicine Website (Accessed November 28, 2012): http://www.faim.org/stemcell/brazziniinstituteasctvideos.html.

19. Xuejun Kong, et al., "Prospects of Stem Cell Therapy for Autism Spectrum Disorders," *North American Journal of Medicine and Science*, vol. 4, no. 3 (July 2011): pp. 134–8.

20. Kathleen Raven, "First US Stem Cell Trial for Autistic Children Launches Today," *Spoonful of Medicine* (posted August 21, 2012, accessed November 29, 2012). Nature Website: http://blogs.nature.com/spoonful/2012/08/first-us-stem-cell-trial-for-autistic-children-launches-today.html.

21. Stem Cells Ecuador Clinic of Treatment and Research Website (accessed November 30, 2012): http://stemcellsecuador.com.

22. "Diabetes Center" Beijing Puhua International Hospital Website (accessed November 29, 2012): http://puhuachina.com.

CHAPTER THIRTEEN

1. R.C. Hell, et al., "Physical activity improves age-related decline in the osteogenic potential of rats' bone marrow-derived mesenchymal stem cells," *Acta Physiologica,* vol. 205, no. 2 (June 2012): pp. 292–301.

2. B. Klotz, et al., "1,25-dihydroxyvitamin D3 treatment delays cellular aging in human mesenchymal stem cells while maintaining their multipotent capacity," *PLoS One,* vol. 7, no. 1 (2012): e. 29959.

CHAPTER FOURTEEN

1. Joseph A. DiMasi, et al., "The Price of Innovation: New Estimates of Drug Development Costs," *Journal of Health Economics,* vol. 22 (2003): pp. 151–85.

2. OCEBM Levels of Evidence Working Group, "The Oxford 2011 Levels of Evidence," Oxford Centre for Evidence-Based Medicine, Website (accessed November 9, 2012): http://www.cebm.net/index.aspx?o=5653.

3. David Rabago, et al., "Hypertonic Dextrose Injections (Prolotherapy) for Knee Osteoarthritis: Results of a Single-arm Uncontrolled Study with 1-year Follow-Up," *Journal of Alternative and Complementary Medicine,* vol. 18, no. 4 (April 2012): pp. 408–14.

4. Gaston Andres Topol, et al., "Hyperosmolar Dextrose Injection for Recalcitrant Osgood-Schlatter Disease," *Pediatrics,* vol. 128, no. 5 (November 2011): pp. E1–E8.

5. Michael Scarpone, et al., "The Efficacy of Prolotherapy for Lateral Epicondylosis: A Pilot Study," *Clinical Journal of Sports Medicine,* vol. 18, no. 3 (May 2008): pp. 248–54.

6. Gaston Andres Topol, "Arthroscopically Monitored Effects of Prolotherapy in Knee Osteoarthritis: Pilot Data," UW Hackett-Hemwall Prolotherapy Research Symposium (Madison, WI.: University of Wisconsin School of Medicine and Public Health, October 20, 2010).

7. Arlette Saenz, "Texas Gov. Rick Perry Received Experimental Stem Cell Therapy," ABCnews.go.com (posted August 4, 2011, accessed December 7, 2012). Website: http://abcnews.go.com/Politics/texas-gov-rick-perry-re-

ceived-experimental-stem-cell/story?id=14232057#.UMJi2IacvIU.

8. Todd Ackerman, "Perry Brings His Stem-cell Cause to Houston," Chron. com (posted October 30, 2012, accessed December 7, 2012).Website: http://www.chron.com/news/houston-texas/houston/article/Perry-brings-Texas-stem-cell-cause-to-Houston-3985899.php.

CHAPTER FIFTEEN

1. R.G. Klein, et al., "Proliferant Injections for Low Back Pain: Histologic Changes of Injected Ligaments and Objective Measures of Lumbar Spine Mobility Before and After Treatment," *Journal of Neurologic Orthopaedic Medicine and Surgery*, vol. 10 (1989): pp. 141–4.

2. R.G. Klein, et al., "A Randomized Double-blind Trial of Dextrose-glycerine-phenol Injections for Chronic, Low Back Pain," *Journal of Spinal Disorders*, vol. 6, no. 1 (1993): pp. 23–33.

3. David Rabago, et al., "A Randomized Controlled Trial of Dextrose Prolotherapy for Knee Osteoarthritis," *Annals of Family Medicine* (2013). In press.

4. David Rabago, et al., "Dextrose Prolotherapy for Knee Osteoarthritis: Results of a Randomized Controlled Trial," *Osteoarthritis and Cartilage*, vol. 19 (2011): pp. S142–3.

5. Ibid.

6. Gaston Andres Topol, et al., "Hyperosmolar Dextrose Injection for Recalcitrant Osgood-Schlatter Disease," *Pediatrics*, vol. 128, no. 5 (November 2011): pp. E1–8.

7. Michael Scarpone, et al., "The Efficacy of Prolotherapy for Lateral Epicondylosis: A Pilot Study," *Clinical Journal of Sports Medicine*, vol. 18, no. 3 (May 2008): pp. 248–54.

8. David Rabago, "David Rabago's Team Takes a Rigorous Look at Prolotherapy for Tennis Elbow," Fammed.wisc.edu (posted January 2012, accessed November 17, 2012). Department of Family Medicine, University of Wisconsin School of Medicine and Public Health Website: http://www.fammed.wisc.edu/our-department/newsletter/winter-2011/prolotherapy-tennis-elbow.

9. Gaston Andres Topol, "Arthroscopically Monitored Effects of Prolotherapy in Knee Osteoarthritis: Pilot Data," UW Hackett-Hemwall Prolotherapy Research Symposium (Madison, WI.: University of Wisconsin School of Medicine and Public Health, October 20, 2010).

10. Young Uck Kim, "Case Reports and Cost Analysis," Anatomy, Diagnosis, and Treatment of Chronic Myofascial Pain with Prolotherapy Research Symposium (Madison, WI: University of Wisconsin School of Medicine and Public Health, October 21–23, 2012).

11. Terri Thompson, "Yankees' Alex Rodriguez's Orthokine Therapy for Knee in Germany Centers on Proteins," NYDailyNews.com (posted December 28, 2011, accessed December 3, 2012).Website: http://www.nydailynews.com/sports/baseball/yankees/ny-yankees-alex-rodriguez-orthokine-therapy-knee-germany-centers-proteins-article-1.998190.

12. Nicholas Kulish, "Novel Blood Treatment Lures Athletes to Germany," *New York Times* (July 11, 2012): p. B12.

13. Simon Dagenais, et al., "Intraligamentous Injections of Sclerosing Solutions (Prolotherapy) for Spinal Pain: A Critical Review of the Literature," *Spine Journal*, vol. 5 (2005): p. 324.

14. All of these rules reference FDA regulation designated 21CFR 1271.1-3.

15. Letter from Ellen F. Lazarus, Director, Division of Human Tissues, Department of Health and Human Services, Food and Drug Administration, to Mitchell S. Fuerst, Esquire (posted November 2011, accessed November 19, 2012). Website: http://box.com/s/v8du7czi944s3xlblr5g.

16. Matthew Herper, "The Truly Staggering Cost of Inventing New Drugs," Forbes.com (posted February 2, 2012, accessed October 15, 2012). Website: http://www.forbes.com/sites/matthewharper/2012/02/22/the-truly-staggering-cost-of-inventing-new-drugs-the-print-version.

17. E. Kon, et al. "Platelet-rich Plasma: Intra-articular Knee Injections Produced Favorable Results on Degenerative Cartilage Lesions," *Knee Surgery, Sports Traumatology, Arthroscopy*, vol. 18, no. 4 (April 2010): pp. 472–9.

ABOUT THE AUTHORS

ABOUT BRIAN J. SHIPLE, D.O.

Brian J. Shiple, D.O., is a recognized leader in the fields of interventional and integrative orthopedic medicine, regenerative injection treatment (RIT), sports medicine, and diagnostic ultrasound. He has been in private practice for six years after completing thirteen years as the division chief of Sports Medicine and director of the Sports Medicine Fellowship Program at one of the major health care systems in the Philadelphia area. He is involved in clinical research and is an active member of various national sports medicine and orthopedic organizations. He teaches nationally and internationally. In the past fifteen years he has spoken at over one hundred conferences and taught RIT to more than 1,000 doctors from eighteen countries.

Dr. Shiple has authored articles and research projects. He has appeared on ESPN and is featured in a PBS show. He was recognized as one of *Philadelphia Magazine's* "Top Docs." Dr. Shiple went on medical service trips to Honduras for seven years, treating underserved people there with prolotherapy while teaching the technique to other doctors from around the world. After being involved in a motor vehicle accident that exacerbated old injuries from playing high school football, Dr. Shiple's chronic injuries almost forced him to leave work and go on disability. His search for effective treatments to help himself ended when he learned about RIT, which saved his career. It has since aided many thousands of his patients.

He holds a Doctor of Osteopathic Medicine degree from the New York College of Osteopathic Medicine and a bachelor's degree in biology from Western Connecticut State University. In addition to having directed the Sports Medicine Fellowship Program at Crozer Keystone, he has taught at the Philadelphia College of Osteopathic Medicine and has held an academic appointment at Temple University School of Medicine. He is a member of the American Osteopathic Association, the American Academy of Family Physicians, the American Medical Society for Sports Medicine, the International Cellular Medicine Society, the American Association of Orthopaedic Medicine, and the International Spine Intervention Society.

He is married and the father of three daughters. Recreationally he is an avid cyclist and also enjoys golf, snow skiing, and scuba diving.

ABOUT MARLISE WABUN WIND, M.S.

Marlise Wabun Wind, M.S., is the author of ten other non-fiction books, with over two million copies in print worldwide in many languages. She holds a master's degree in journalism from Columbia University and a bachelor's degree in international communications from George Washington University. She is a lifelong student of cross-cultural healing, complementary and holistic medicine, and wellness. One of her books is about integrative healing, and several others are about cross-cultural healing techniques, comparative philosophies, religions and spirituality. Ms. Wind was searching for an alternative to the surgical treatments for an arthritic ankle when she was referred to Dr. Shiple, and it was through him that she learned about RIT.

Ms. Wind resides in the Greater Philadelphia area with her husband. Thomas Wind, D.O. is a child, adolescent, and adult psychiatrist who does therapy, evaluations, medication management, and research. He is knowledgeable about a wide range of integrative medicine. He was always available to explain medical concepts and terms while Marlise was working on this book. Managing Thomas's practice and understanding his schedule were helpful in working with Dr. Shiple, since both men are exceptionally busy, compassionate physicians.

Marlise and Thomas are the parents of Kyla, a talented, hard-working artist and a superb communicator, teacher, and nurturer. She received a B.A. from Ursinus College in Collegeville, Pennsylvania, and completed post-baccalaureate work in studio art at the Pennsylvania Academy of Fine Arts.

Marlise Wind is currently working on several other projects, including a novel and a spiritual adventure memoir, as well as four other non-fiction titles concerning ceremony and celebrations, relationships, parenting healthy children, and what she is calling "mother sense." Because of her own knowledge of the physical limitations of arthritis and pain, she is an informal medical advocate for friends who need such support. She has lectured widely about all of the aforementioned topics and is available for speaking and workshops.

INDEX

avascular necrosis (AVN), 183–85, 314–15

B

back pain
  case reports
    prolotherapy, 15–16, 124–25, 128–31, 133–35, 206–7, 219–21
    PRP, 206–7
    PSI, 141–43, 144
  causes of, 86, 91–92
  conventional treatment of, 49–50
  treatment selection considerations, 8, 107–8
Bankart lesions, 213
bare foot running, 93
B-complex vitamins, 253, 257
biomechanical assessments, 90, 104
biopuncture, 153–54
bisphosphonates, 255, 261
blastomeric stem cells, 173
bleeding, risk of, 261–62, 305
blood, clotting of, 158, 159–60, 240–41
blood flow, 162, 241, 256
blood pressure medications, 255
body, symmetry/asymmetry of, 78–79, 90
body building, 199–200
bone death, 314–15
bone marrow
  oxygen levels in, 252–53
  as source of stem cells, 174, 178, 297, 303, 307
  transplantation of, 263
bone spurs, 126, 220–21
Born to Run (McDougall), 93
bovine collagen, 178
bracing and support, 88–90, 188, 259–60

business model, of health care, 83

C

calcaneous fractures, 220
calcitonin gene-related peptide (CGRP), 140
calorie restriction, 250
cardiovascular health, 63–64, 158, 194
cartilage
  injuries to, 302. *See also* meniscal tears
  regeneration of, 192, 211–12, 283–84
  supplements for, 252–53
  types of, 182
case reports, purpose of, 275–76
casts and casting, 88
Cayman Island Regenexx Clinic, 193, 307–8, 313
Celebrex, 63–64, 242
Centeno, Christopher, 159
centrifuge systems, 263, 280, 288
CGRP (calcitonin gene-related peptide), 140
children
  autism study, 194
  RIT treatment suitability, 132
  sports injuries in, 55, 113–14, 229–30
chiropractic medicine, 79, 82, 142, 243
"chocolate bar test," 250
chondral lesions, 302–3
chondroitin, 241, 242, 253, 256
chronic ankle instability, 53
chronic injuries
  defined, 34, 217

I

treatment selection considerations, 8

knee replacement surgery, 3, 54, 234–35

Koop, C. Everett, 2, 120–21

L

labral tears
  case reports, 203–4, 213
  extent of, 302–3
laser therapy, 94
lateral epicondylitis. *See* tennis elbow
lateral femoral cutaneous nerve, entrapment of, 227–28
legal issues. *See* insurance coverage; litigation; regulatory issues
leg length differences, 91–92
leg pain, 8, 9
lidocaine
  with ASCI, 238, 260–61
  in biopuncture, 153
  in nerve blocks, 70
  pain management role, 305–6
  in prolotherapy, 118, 121
  in PSI, 139, 141
  in trigger point therapy, 85
lifestyle considerations, 104–5, 133–35
Ligagenix, 241, 252, 253, 256
ligaments
  injuries to. *See also specific injuries/ligaments*
  conventional treatments for, 3
  extent of tears, 291–92
  reconstruction recovery times, 122–23
  RIT treatment suitability, 117, 213–14
  laxity/looseness in, 80–81, 198–99,

235
listening, importance of, 47–48
litigation, 133, 268, 298–99
low-carb diets, 249–51
lubricants, viscosupplement injections as, 70
Lyftogt, John, 139, 140, 149

M

malpractice suits, 268, 298–99
manganese, 253, 256
manipulation, in osteopathic medicine, 78–82
marijuana use, 257
massage, 97, 244. *See also* myofascial release muscle manipulation
McDougall, Christopher, 93
medial collateral ligament (MCL), 205
medial epicondylitis, 215
medical awareness, of patients, 103–4, 110–13, 127–28, 322–23
medical equipment, testing of, 38, 284–85. *See also* drug testing
Medicare coverage, 121
medications. *See also* drug testing
  antibiotics, 65–67, 147–48, 255, 261
  contraindications, with RIT, 176, 240, 242, 246, 254–55, 261–62, 292–93
  for pain
    adverse effects on healing, 11–12, 49, 53, 61–69, 118
    caused by RIT, 122, 179, 190, 305–6
    hormone interactions, 190, 224
    reflex inhibition effects, 45–47
  stem cell classification as, 299, 317
  steroids

S